SITREP

12/23/02

To Bea and Paul,

I had support from
many "families", but the
original family is the best.
Go USA!

Larry Wannefelts

SITREP

◆

E-mails from the Front Lines of the Cancer War

Larry Warrenfeltz

Writer's Showcase
San Jose New York Lincoln Shanghai

SITREP
E-mails from the Front Lines of the Cancer War

Writer's Showcase
an imprint of iUniverse, Inc.

For information address:
iUniverse, Inc.
5220 S. 16th St., Suite 200
Lincoln, NE 68512
www.iuniverse.com

ISBN: 0-595-24101-8

For the Lovely Nurse Nancy. Life wouldn't be worthwhile without you—and I wouldn't be here to enjoy it.

"Never give up. Don't EVER give up!"
—Jim Valvano

Contents

Acknowledgements

If it were physically possible to remember and recognize everyone who deserves thanks for helping Nancy and me win this particular battle of the cancer wars, I would need a separate volume. The kind words, thoughts, acts, cards, e-mails, gifts, phone calls, jokes, and most of all—the prayers—were the nourishment on which we fed for six months.

They came from all around the world. They came from people we had known well for many, many years and from people we had just met. They came from people we hadn't talked to in years, and even from people we have never met! The best part was that they were all heartfelt expressions from humans reaching out to try to help another person in their time of need. It strengthened my determination and reassured me of the basic goodness of people.

I often wonder if the level of support would have been as amazing before September 11th. It probably would not have been. The terrorist attacks drew us closer, made us more sensitive to others, and more willing to reach out to help someone else. If that's the case, then I willingly accept my good fortune. I hope we maintain our improved manners and our increased concern for others. It sure makes my world a nicer place to live.

The Lovely Nurse Nancy is way at the top of my list of folks to thank. Throughout surgery, chemo, recovery, and survivorship my wife has been an indomitable tower of strength. I'm not surprised, because she's been a 5'4", 110-pound endless source of love and encouragement ever since we met. She never let her positive attitude slip. She endured my mood swings, periods of no communication beyond moans and grunts, and my endless demands without ever losing her good humor. I can't imagine tackling any difficult task without her. Beating cancer would have been impossible.

Jim and Lindsay were naturally worried about Dad, but they balanced their lives well enough to continue their excellence in school while occasionally checking with me by phone, e-mail, or instant messaging.

Our families are far away, but the phone calls made it seem like they were close by. I still feel bad about refusing to talk to you, Mom. Thanks for understanding!

Here is a partial list of people to whom I owe my health, my thanks, and my prayers:

- The medical teams at the Pensacola Naval Hospital, Sacred Heart Hospital, and Hematology and Oncology Associates were superb, especially Dr. Mike Schneider and Dr. Thomas Tan.

- The staff on 4-West—y'all are the best!

- A huge thanks to my Cancer Coaches—Cheryl Shank and Cynthia Bassich. It takes a survivor to really understand.

- Special thanks to all the other cancer warriors and spouses who willingly shared their stories, advice, and support—Jim Bassich, Mitch Shank, Leslie, Don, Mike, Bob, Nancy, Matt, Carol, Steve, Auntie Muriel, Dave, Patti, Rick, Brad, Jerry, Randy, Deborah and many more.

- Ty, Charlie, Stacy, and Kelly—the best friends in the world.

- Billie and Jeff, FJ and Bob, Julie and Jeff, Maria(h) and Pete

- Kathy and Ray ("It's great to be a Dad!")

- Carl June—cancer expert in too many ways

- Paul Gaffney

- Linda and Rob

- Ken Ford, Tim Wright, Jack Hansen, and the IHMCers

- The Littletons
- Nancy and Tim, Alex and Terry, Sheila 'Mac' and Bob
- Brian and Gillian, Sean and Tara, Don and Jane, Blake and Terri
- Rich and Debbie
- Ed and Michelle, Dave and Chiyoko
- Tami, Cindie, and the Argonauts
- Ronette (and your mom and dad)
- Lisa Frailey and Tim Rush—purveyors of fine Italian candy
- Sallie and Ken, Becky and Mike
- Bruce—"God Bless America and Let's Play Ball"
- "LIMDU Connie"
- Les Raske
- Pam Long
- Phil and Brian, who set a new record at the BCNR
- Chick Chikanovich—the Surgeon General of Laughter
- Burdman—artist extraordinaire
- Pat Smith
- My NAVO family

Go USA!

1

Nobody Volunteers for This War

On the morning of Tuesday September 11, 2001 I awoke to a pair of interns huddled around the foot of my bed and removing the bandages from my right ankle. I had been operated on the evening before at the Naval Hospital in Pensacola, Florida to clean out an area of skin cancer.

On the day before, my scheduled time for non-emergency surgery had come and gone while my wife and I waited for the weekend rush of quasi-emergency cases to be treated. It was after dinnertime before they finally put me under and went to work. I vaguely remembered getting wheeled out of the recovery room and into my room on the hospital ward just before halftime of the Monday night football game. I have no idea who won or even who was playing.

By 6:00 am Tuesday I was still in a bit of an anesthetic haze and under the influence of strong intravenous painkillers. I raised my hospital bed to see what was going on. As the last layers of gauze came off I saw an open surgical wound that was a whole lot bigger than I expected. It stretched six inches from just above my ankle to my lower calf and wrapped all the way around the inside half of my leg. I recognized my anklebone and Achilles tendon. I quickly lay the bed back down and never looked at it again. My cancer war, for which I had not volunteered, was going to be a whole lot more than a skirmish.

Less than two hours later our entire world and all of our lives changed. America and our allies were thrust into a war we didn't want, and it was far more intense than we expected. **9/11/01** carries strong emotional memories for every American. You know where you were and what you were doing when you heard about the terrorist attacks. Unless you were completely out of touch with civilization on that day, you watched the news coverage in a state of shock. Most of us remember the horror as we watched the second plane full of innocent civilians strike the south tower of the World Trade Center.

Lying captive in a hospital bed, the day was surreal for me. My mind flickered back and forth between my unanticipated personal cancer war and the new World War on Terrorism. I had been knocked off my feet in both. It was the beginning of a dual battle against the terrorist cells—one set hidden in locations around the world, the other set microscopic within my body. One war was fought on a global stage while the other was confined between the covers of a thick medical record. Over the coming months I was reminded again and again of the parallels between the two fights.

◆   ◆   ◆

As the days grew shorter at the end of the summer of 2001, I had reached the end of a 26-year career as a Sailor in the United States Navy. When you include the four years I spent at the U.S. Naval Academy in Annapolis, I had spent my entire adult life from age 17 to 48 on active duty. Needless to say, cancer surgery was not how I had planned to begin my life after the Navy. Over the years I thought I had learned to expect the unexpected and adapt to change as it developed, but a personal medical emergency blind-sided me. The diagnosis of cancer shook my family and me deeply.

In our 24-year marriage, my wife Nancy and I had made friends around the world. Many were Navy people. Many others were the "civilians" we got to know along the way. In California, Virginia, Louisiana, Italy, and everywhere else we were stationed, Nancy hung a plaque in her kitchen with the inscription "Home is Where the Navy

Sends You." Wherever we were stationed, she made it a happy home for our family. Our post-Navy strategy was to send ourselves to a new home in the Florida Panhandle and enjoy a new life and a new career.

Over the years, our friends scattered all around the world. A few of them knew I had been diagnosed with skin cancer, but many didn't. Some people heard rumors that were only loosely related to the facts. I thought it was important to let people hear about it directly from me, rather than receive a distorted version through the Coconut Telegraph. We planned to spread the accurate word using Internet e-mails.

◆   ◆   ◆

Going into the surgery, we had what I thought was a very good plan of attack. The surgeon, Major Michael Schneider, USAF, would perform a wide area excision to clean out any remains of a small tumor that he had removed two weeks earlier. He would also use dye and radioactive markers to mark the lymph nodes in my right groin that drained the ankle area. He would remove the sentinel nodes so we could see if the cancer had spread to other areas. At the end of the operation, the surgeons would close the wound with a skin graft from my left thigh. I expected to be in the hospital about 48 hours.

During surgery, Doctor Mike found that the cancer in my ankle area was more extensive than we originally thought. There were four satellite tumors near the primary site. To get a clean margin, he removed much more tissue than he expected. He and his colleagues in the operating room decided to leave the wound open rather than do an immediate skin graft. There were several benefits to that decision. My body immediately started generating granulation tissue to fill in the sizeable hole. It also allowed the option of relatively simple additional surgery in case the terrorist cells had spread their poison even farther than my doctors estimated during my time on the operating table.

The down side to leaving the large surgical wound open was that I now required three-times-a-day dressing changes. Each change was a

major operation. It meant rubber gloves, a sterile field, a pile of dressings, rolls of gauze, protective pads, a bag to hold all the trash, and
more than just a little pain. The wet-to-dry dressing technique started
with saline-saturated dressings next to the wound with layers of dry
gauze over top. But wet or dry, peeling the dressing from the open
wound hurt—a lot. For the next two weeks my favorite words from the
corpsmen were, "OK, Captain. It's all off."

I never even considered asking Nancy to do the dressing changes.
She's good at just about everything that you want a wife and mother to
be good at, including nursing husband and children through the typical family maladies. But I knew she didn't want to look at that wound
any more than I did. So we decided that wound care and pain manage-
ment would keep me at the Naval Hospital for the foreseeable future.
As Doctor Mike said, at that point we were planning about a half-day
at a time.

◆   ◆   ◆

Fortunately, in July of 2001, I had started my post-Navy career
doing research administration for the University of West Florida's
Institute for Human and Machine Cognition. The Cognition Institute
is blessed with visionary leaders that stand right up there with the finest
Naval officers I know. I can't think of higher praise. Even though I had
only been working for them for a few weeks, Ken Ford, Tim Wright,
and Jack Hansen made sure that I knew they fully supported me in my
war.

When I realized I was going to be stuck in the hospital for several
weeks, I called the Institute and asked them if they could set up my
laptop computer so I could dial in to their server. Nancy picked it up
later that day and I was soon wired to the Internet.

There were messages from many friends offering support, love,
thoughts and prayers. Nancy and I decided that once we received the
results from the pathology lab's look at the tissues from the operation, I

would send out a situation report to my various address lists. She would then forward it to all of her friends. As it turned out, friends relayed the news to other mutual acquaintances, who then sent it onward. We soon had a prayer chain that wrapped all the way around the world.

SITREP #1

9/15/01

Dear Family, Friends, Shipmates, and Co-workers,

What a strange and horrible week our country has just endured. However, I'm now firmly convinced that the terrorists made a terrible mistake. Our country and our world will end up far better in the long run, despite their barbaric efforts.

But I can't personally do much in the war on terrorism (just yet). I have to continue my personal war against a nasty and rare bugger of a skin cancer called Merkle cell carcinoma. This past Monday we attacked it by removing a rather hefty chunk of the inside of my right lower leg. (I'm going to tell people I was surfing amongst the "square-mouth" sharks of the Gulf of Mexico.) At the same time, we found evidence that the cancer is moving through the lymph system, as it typically does. Before it gets a chance to set up shop in other locations in my body, we'll hit it with a course of chemotherapy. That starts Monday at Sacred Heart hospital in Pensacola. At this point, I don't know how long the chemotherapy will last.

We aren't positive what we'll do after the chemo—maybe radiation, and certainly some more lymph and leg biopsies, a skin graft to cover the "shark bite," and lots of prayers for complete annihilation of the enemy.

Yesterday I read Lance Armstrong's book, "It's Not About the Bike." To refresh your memory, Armstrong defeated long odds to survive cancer, and has since won three consecutive Tours de France—some say the toughest athletic competition in the world. He received an e-mail just after he announced his cancer that said, "You don't know it yet, but we're the lucky ones." Lance now agrees. I look forward to learning the lesson for myself. To quote Lance, "If you asked me to choose between winning the Tour de France and cancer, I would choose cancer. Odd as it sounds, I would rather have the title cancer survivor than winner of the Tour."

Thank you, everyone for your tremendous love and support. Your thoughts and prayers are key parts of our battle plan. Please keep 'em coming. I love hearing from folks!

Go Navy, Army, Air Force, Marines, Coast Guard! Go USA! Larry

2

What the Hell is Merkle Cell?

On Friday September 14, Doctor Schneider came to see me with the reports from the pathology laboratory. Of course, I wanted him to say that we had caught the tumor in time to cut it all out while it was still confined to the ankle area. But knowing the nature of my particular type of cancer, I was prepared for the worst. The news wasn't good. Of the five lymph nodes he had removed, four were positive. (Well, I suppose that's better than five for five!) Also, there were microscopic cancerous cells in the upper edge of the leg wound.

Mike had done a lot of research on the Internet, and had consulted with experts around the country. There was no doubt in our mind what we had to do—attack! And we would follow Colin Powell's doctrine. We would go after a specific objective with overwhelming force and have a clear exit strategy. Chemotherapy was our weapon of choice.

◆　　　◆　　　◆

I had first noticed a small lump on the inside of my right leg a few inches above the ankle during the spring of 2001. I didn't think anything about it. Since my Little League days, I have spent a whole lot of my time on baseball and softball fields. For years my shins and legs had regularly taken a beating as Lindsay, my fastpitch softball superstar daughter, perfected her drop and change up. I also enjoy umpiring, and I have spent many hours behind the plate where my too small shin guards didn't always adequately protect my too long legs. The lump didn't even hurt, and didn't appear to be growing.

There was a lot happening in our lives in the first half of 2001. Lindsay, the younger of our two children, graduated from high school in May. I was ready to make the transition from a lifetime of active duty naval service into a second career. After several months of testing the civilian employment waters, I accepted an offer from the Cognition Institute. We were preparing to put our house in Louisiana on the market so we could move to Florida. We entertained a number of houseguests and enjoyed a seemingly continuous round of dinners and parties. My health in general, and the small lump on my leg in particular, were not high on the list of things demanding my attention.

We held a memorable Navy retirement ceremony the same week Lindsay graduated from Fontainebleau High School in Mandeville, Louisiana. We planned it that way so visiting family could be present to witness both of our big days. I had spent my last six years in the Navy assigned to three different jobs at the Stennis Space Center in south Mississippi, just a few miles from the Louisiana border. We enjoyed our time in our big house in the St. Tammany Parish suburb across Lake Pontchartrain from New Orleans.

In January of her senior year, Lindsay verbally committed to play softball for the Argonauts of the University of West Florida. She signed a partial scholarship in April. Her brother Jim had graduated from Fontainebleau two years before Lindsay. He took advantage of a full-tuition academic scholarship to Tulane University and even raked in three additional scholarships that went a long way toward covering his room and board. He was happy at Tulane, doing well in his studies, and was dating a wonderful Tulane classmate.

As impending empty nesters with a decent retirement check guaranteed to arrive every month, Nancy and I were free agents. Ever since I had earned a doctorate in meteorology in 1987, I had occasionally dreamed of going to work in a college atmosphere. I was confident that

I could find a position in the academic world. We only had to decide whether we wanted to stay in Louisiana or look elsewhere.

We decided it was time to make one more move. The question was where? Nancy recalled that every time we had visited the Florida Panhandle, we would look at each other and say, "Wouldn't it be nice to live here?" I focused my job search on Florida. We figured that a house there would be a good way to lure our families from Pennsylvania, Maryland, and West Virginia (and even my brother Lon in south Florida) to visit us in the Panhandle.

I accepted the job at UWF just days before my retirement ceremony and announced my new career plans at my retirement dinner. I then set about using all the leave I had accumulated over the last several years of active duty. Including a couple of weeks off for job hunting and house hunting, I had enough time saved up to stretch my actual retirement date to September 1st. I started work at UWF and rented a one-bedroom furnished apartment in Pensacola. Nancy put our Louisiana house on the market and started shopping for a new home in Florida, while continuing her part time job at a cool Mandeville toy store—The Magic Box. I drove the three-hour trip back and forth along Interstate 10 almost every weekend.

Between the new job, the old house, and travel softball, July went by in a blur. I slept in eight different beds in four different states, and nowhere more than five nights in a row. I was one of the assistant coaches of Lindsay's summer softball team, the Louisiana High Voltage. The Volts qualified for the American Fastpitch Association National Tournament in Beaumont, Texas. Lindsay and I spent a week there with the team beginning July 30. We won four games before we were eliminated. It was an emotional and memorable capstone to her six-year High Voltage career. At our farewell meeting, I told the team that if I were ever in the position to hire people, I would look for travel softball players. Those young ladies learn the value of dedication, hard work, and teamwork while still in their teens.

◆   ◆   ◆

Through the summer, the lump on my leg bugged me. It didn't hurt, and it did not appear to be changing, but it wasn't going away, either. When I returned to Pensacola after the Nationals, I decided to get it checked out. I figured it would be a lot easier to go to Sick Call as an active duty captain than to get in line for treatment with the rest of the retirees, so I wanted to do it in August, before my September 1st transfer to the retired list. The doctor at Sick Call referred me to the surgery clinic.

On Friday August 17, I met with Dr. Mike Schneider. He suspected a harmless cyst or a fatty lipoma, but recommended we cut it out. We walked down to an outpatient surgery room. While he numbed my leg and cut out the lump we had a nice conversation about my new job and how an Air Force surgeon ended up assigned to the Navy Hospital. "Have a great weekend!"

The following Tuesday, Mike reached me on my cell phone. I had liked his style from the first time I met him. He is young, energetic, and confident. (Nancy adds, "…and good-looking, too.") He's absolutely honest and doesn't pull any punches.

He told me, "That thing was malignant, and I don't know what it is. When can you come in?"

The first priority was to get a chest X-ray. It was clear. The pathology folks still hadn't figured out what kind of cancer I had. Mentally, the time we spent waiting to find out (whoever heard of leg cancer?) was the toughest eight days of the whole war. Mike scheduled a CT scan and a complete upper and lower endoscopy.

The preliminary results of the CT scan were good. Now, an endoscopy requires a completely clear digestive system. That means fasting for a day then taking a couple of doses of stuff that makes you "blow tubes," in Navy terms.

Mike called the afternoon of my fast. He asked, "You didn't take that stuff yet, did you?"

"Not yet," I answered.

"Well don't. The Armed Forces Institute of Pathology ID'd your case as a rare type of skin cancer called Merkle cell carcinoma."

To celebrate the relatively good news, Nancy and I had dinner at McGuires Irish Pub rather than suffering through an evening of clear liquids.

◆   ◆   ◆

There have only been about 600 documented cases of Merkle cell carcinoma. If you research the statistics, they aren't very good. Once it reaches the lymph system, it metastasizes rapidly and turns deadly. We decided from the beginning that we weren't concerned with the percentages. Every cancer warrior is a case study of one. You either win or you don't. Besides, I was at least two decades younger than the average Merkle cell warrior and I suspect I was in much better condition overall.

With cancer evident in the lymph system, we had to assume it had a clear path to spread anywhere in my body. We now had the intelligence proof that tied my terrorist cells to a small but deadly organization. Like Osama bin Laden's al-Qaeda, it appeared to be well organized and vicious. But like al-Qaeda, it was in reality a misguided aberration—an abnormal growth that grabbed a base of operations and needed to be totally eliminated. Chemotherapy was our choice. We needed a systemic weapon that would find the cancer cells and kill them—regardless of where they were hidden.

3

Oncology Foxholes

SITREP #2

9/16/01

Dear Family, Friends, Classmates, Shipmates, Argonauts, IHMCers, et al.,

Nothing new on the medical scene, but I just had to share this:

Sometimes we ask God for a "sign." In my prayers I've asked for strength and courage, but not specifically for a sign. But consider this…

This morning I watched ABC's talking heads recapping the horrible events of this week. Cokie Roberts was interviewing Attorney General John Ashcroft. Behind him was a view of a small, peaceful town with lots of trees and a pretty brick church. I realized it was my hometown of Smithsburg, MD. The press corps headquarters to cover Camp David is set up in my high school. The church is Trinity Lutheran, where I grew up.

Physically, I've got a tough battle ahead. Mentally, I'm in the absolute best shape of my life—and that is the absolute truth.

Go USA! Larry

I grew up in an active Lutheran household. We didn't miss church. Mom taught Sunday school and sang in the choir. My Dad, herding his four sons down the center aisle, took over the third pew from the front, on the left side of Trinity Lutheran Church in the little town of Smithsburg. My parents were born, raised, and still live there. I love taking my family back to Trinity whenever we visit, even though our seats aren't "reserved" anymore.

Smithsburg is a map dot surrounded by small farms and orchards in beautiful western Maryland. It's right where Pennsylvania and West

Virginia squeeze Maryland down to a scant few miles. My youngest brother Daryl lives in Waynesboro, PA. He and his wife and kids can drive to my parents' house in ten minutes. Brother Dean lives with his family in Martinsburg, WV—25 minutes away. Brother number three is Lon, who lives with his family in Naples, on south Florida's Gulf Coast. I am the oldest of the four.

When I was in school, Smithsburg's population climbed upward all the way past 500. Most of my classmates came to Smithsburg High School on buses from the farms, from the surrounding even-smaller villages, or from Fort Ritchie, a small Army post on South Mountain just east of town.

Also on the ridge of South Mountain are several beautiful parks and an unmarked, well-hidden compound called Camp David. I remember one Sunday when President Lyndon and Lady Bird Johnson drove to Smithsburg to attend the Episcopal Church right behind our house. The president drove himself through town in a big powder-blue convertible. We junior high students were terribly insulted when the *Washington Post* society columnist lamented that Lady Bird could only show off her spring finery to the "country bumpkins."

Seeing Smithsburg on national television that September Sunday morning is easy to explain. It's a beautiful setting, and the press corps was already there. President Bush had gathered key advisors at Camp David to plan strategy for the war on terrorism. When Mom called, she said the fighters flying combat air patrol kept them awake the night before. Nevertheless, the town had never been showcased on national television before. I was alone in my hospital room when I saw the church. I'm not smart enough to know if it was "a sign from God," but it sure did make me feel better!

Jamie Burd is a Naval Academy classmate ('75 Sir!) who retired after a career in the Navy and revealed a wonderful talent as an artist. After the Burdman got SITREP number two, he got in his car in Annapolis and drove two hours to Smithsburg. He sketched Trinity, then painted the church in watercolor, framed it, and sent it to me. It was one of the most touching things anyone ever did for me. But it was only one of the many thoughtful acts Nancy and I experienced. I guess finding out how many great friends we have is one of the good things that make cancer warriors the "lucky ones."

◆   ◆   ◆

There's an old saying that there are no atheists in foxholes. In my experience, you won't find many sitting in the recliners in the oncologist's office either. Lance Armstrong says anyone who's ever heard the words "*You have cancer*," and thought, "*I'm going to die*" immediately becomes a member of the cancer community. Once you're in it, you never leave. And once you're in it, you instantly begin to learn a whole lot more about yourself. You are immediately much more aware of your own mortality. My natural response was to seek comfort in prayer.

The first prayer to enter my mind when I found out that I had cancer was a verse from Isaiah that my mother copied in the front of my bible when I left home for the Naval Academy in 1971. It has been a source of comfort and strength for me for my entire life.

For I, the Lord your God hold your right hand; it is I who say to you, "Fear not, I will help you."

I've always prayed—formal prayers in church and grace before meals, but more often my prayers are short and informal. I call them "thought prayers." Many times I don't even take the time to put them in the form of words. (I figure God doesn't lower our prayer grades based on our limited vocabulary or poor pronunciation.) When I was in school, I always asked God to help me keep a clear head during tests. I do the same now before important briefings and presentations. I often say to myself, "God, what a beautiful day!" To me, that's a better prayer than one I recite without thinking about the meaning of the words.

I never prayed for a miracle. I do believe in miracles, but I don't believe in asking for them. If God wants to perform a miracle, He will pick the spot. I will ask God for the strength and courage to do whatever I have to do to meet the worldly challenges of the day. So far, that prayer has always been answered. "Thank God!"

◆   ◆   ◆

Nancy is Roman Catholic. She and her mother both keep a supply of Saint Peregrine medals and prayer cards for friends who become cancer warriors. St. Peregrine is the patron saint of cancer patients. I found it fascinating that Peregrine suffered from cancer of the leg! He was miraculously cured the day before he was to have his foot amputated.

Now I personally believe that I don't need a priest or a saint to intercede on my behalf. I know I can go right to the Top Three on my own. But if someone gets a priest, a saint, or the Pope himself to pray on my behalf, I thankfully accept. Our friends cover all the faiths of the spiritual spectrum. They prayed for me according to their own beliefs. We welcomed every kind thought and every prayer.

Some of the St. Peregrine prayer cards call us cancer victims, but I absolutely hate that label. Don Juan wrote that the difference between an ordinary man and a warrior is that the warrior looks at every thing that happens to him as a challenge, while the ordinary man accepts everything as either a blessing or a curse. I'm sure that some cancer patients allow themselves to be victims, but the ones I know are warriors.

◆   ◆   ◆

The chaplains and volunteers in the Pensacola Naval Hospital chaplain's office were available every day to pray, talk, listen, and support us patients and our families. I enjoyed talking with them, but my favorite person at the hospital is a custodial worker named Kenneth. He is a man of God. He cleans the hospital to support his family, but his energy and passion go to his true calling as the pastor of a fundamentalist Baptist church in town. As he worked, Kenneth and I had quite a few discussions about our religious beliefs. I looked forward to the times he would come to my room. He is well read, well spoken, and convincing, but never tried to force me to accept his ideas. We agreed to disagree on creation and evolution. But Kenneth helped me clarify my thoughts on the relationship between God and humans. I hope he knows that the work he did in room 53 on ward 4-West covered a whole lot more than sanitary floors and a clean sink.

Nancy and I saw Kenneth again, a few months later. The night before I began chemo cycle #4, I was depressed and in a bad mood. Cycle 3 had hit me hard, and I was dreading the next round. We drove from Mandeville back to Pensacola for another week in my dreary apartment. Both of us were kind of down, so we decided on the spur of the moment to treat ourselves to a chili and Frosty dinner at Wendy's. We drove to the restaurant, got in line, and there in front of us was Kenneth in his suit and tie, picking up a quick bite after Sunday evening services. Did God or coincidence put us in line together? I don't really care. I do know that seeing Kenneth lifted my spirits and I felt a surge of strength and confidence. A sign from God? An answer to my prayers for strength? I can't say. But I do know for certain that I it sure made me feel better.

◆   ◆   ◆

I was raised to believe that God is omnipotent, omniscient, and a caring and loving God. You know something? You can pick any two of the three, but all three can't possibly be true. At least, they can't be true when you study the problem from our very limited human perspective.

If a caring and loving God knew everything and had the power to prevent bad things from happening, then we wouldn't have airplanes full of innocent people knocking down great buildings. Hard working mailroom employees wouldn't die of anthrax. Babies would never be killed by drunk drivers! The Holocaust would never have happened! But bad things happen to innocent people every single day. In his wonderful book, *When Bad Things Happen to Good People*, Harold Kushner writes of a God who has limited His own power over human interactions. He is loving. He is caring. He knows that we suffer. But by His rules for the universe (which I certainly don't claim to understand) He doesn't allow Himself the power to heal everyone or deliver us from every evil.

Just as God has chosen to limit His omnipotence in human lives, He has given us the responsibility to make our own choices. I don't believe that our entire lives are pre-ordained according to some great master plan. God gave man the ability to make decisions. We don't act according to instinct, as the animals do. We have to make choices. We aren't actors in some huge eternal play in which God has written all the lines and assigned all stage directions. We're more like the players in the old electronic football games. God lines us all up, turns on the power, and we shake and jiggle to our own decisions until the power goes off again.

That's enough of my amateur theology. As I said, once you're a cancer warrior, you learn a lot about yourself. You can pray for strength, courage, patience, and hope. You'll probably have your prayers answered. But you can't expect God to fight the battle for you. You have to make the decision for yourself.

4

Opening a Second Front

SITREP #3

9/17/01

Dear Family, Friends, Shipmates, Classmates, Argonauts, and IHMCers,

Well, I have a new address—Sacred Heart Hospital in Pensacola. The current plan is to stay here for about three days to take the first strong course of chemotherapy. Unfortunately, this room only has one phone line, so I have to cut off the phone to go on-line. If you try to call and get a busy signal, please understand.

It's time to go kick some butt on this cancer!

GO USA! Larry

The Naval Hospital in Pensacola doesn't have an oncology department, so they arranged for me to be transferred to Sacred Heart Hospital for the first round of chemotherapy. When the terrorist cells first struck at me, it was in my ankle. We countered that attack with aggressive surgery. Now the war shifted to the microscopic cells that may (or may not) have still been free in my lymph and circulatory system. Mike had contacted several oncologists in the area. Dr. Thomas Tan was familiar with Merkle cell carcinomas, and was willing to take over as commander of the fight. Dr. Mike was still in charge of what was now the "second front" on my leg.

SITREP #4

9/18/01

Dear Family, Friends, Shipmates, Classmates, Argonauts, and IHMCers,

I just observed a moment of silence with many of you. One week ago this minute our world changed forever. But the healing and strengthening are happening…way ahead of schedule. Our country is going back to basic values and will emerge so much, much stronger. It is a painful way to accomplish it, but the long-term results will be wonderful. I watched the Opening Ceremonies of the Cardinal game in St. Louis while we were waiting to meet the oncologist last night. (Somehow, it's easier to keep the TV on ESPN versus QVC when the nurse call button and the TV remote are on the same unit.) By the time they played God Bless the USA, and sang the National Anthem, and Jack Buck read his poem, the neck of my hospital gown was soaked with tears of pride.

As for me, the healing process is progressing as well. The chemotherapy plan looks like this: six courses (each taking three consecutive days of chemo) spaced out 3–4 weeks apart. That takes us through New Years at least. The first chemo treatment was overnight last night. No adverse effects noticed so far. The hair (what there was) is still there, and thank God, no nausea. Of course, the side effects don't typically show up early—only after you start building up a level of chemicals in your body and tissues. Advances in anti-nausea drugs will help keep that problem manageable, and the hair is no big deal. I had an "easy access" Mediport inserted under the skin below my left collarbone yesterday. Now when it's chemo or other IV time, it's just "plug-and-play." Kind of like having a private DSL line right into the veins. I nicknamed my IV stand "Osama." It's tall, skinny, ugly, and nasty.

Now that we've got that top priority (chemo) penciled-in on the calendar, we'll be able to figure out what to do about the "shark bite" wound above the right ankle. I'm told it is healing nicely. (I'm too much of a wimp to look.)

Thanks for the hundreds of e-mails and phone calls. I'm sorry I don't have time to answer all the e-mails, but I read and appreciate every one. I certainly have some creative and funny friends. That you are also supportive, patriotic, and wonderful goes without saying.

GO USA! Larry

The three days I spent as a patient at Sacred Heart all run together as a blur in my memory. I found later that chemotherapy has that effect. I call it "chemo-brain." I know that I was released from the Naval Hospital and taken to Sacred Heart. After a week of nothing but air conditioning and hospital smells, I remember the joy of feeling the warm, humid outside air as the Navy paramedics moved the gurney from the ambulance to the door of the new hospital. I remember worrying that Nancy would have a hard time finding Sacred Heart. She hadn't been in Pensacola very long, and the time she had spent there was mostly with me. I know she eventually tracked me down and that we waited for a long time to meet my new doctor.

Dr. Tan is a hard-working oncologist who puts in amazingly long hours. He always takes time to really listen and talk to all of his patients. His office manager told me many months later that she has the phrase "...after a lengthy discussion..." programmed into her computer for when she transcribes Dr. Tan's consultation notes. As a result, he's almost always running behind schedule and late for appointments. But I would rather have a doctor who is obviously concerned about his patients instead of one who cuts off your visit when you are still pondering questions and concerns. Dr. Tan came in to see us late that evening.

After a quick check of my heart and lungs, we started talking about my cancer and how we would attack it. He had the same sobering statistics on Merkle cell tumors that Dr. Schneider had given me earlier. But he quickly adopted my personal theory that I was going to be a case study of one person, and that the averages weren't applicable. He explained the treatment protocol he recommended, along with the probable side effects, and the schedule for the six cycles of chemotherapy. All in all, it was a confidence-building meeting.

Dr. Schneider had installed the mediport, or "vascular access device," the morning I left the Naval Hospital. It is an ingenious device that provides direct access to a major vein in your chest. It meant no more IV sticks. Even for a relatively young person with good veins, a long period on an IV is a problem. The IV site has to be changed every couple of days, and there are only so many places on your hands and wrists that can be used. Before he installed my port, Mike asked on which side I wanted it situated. He always asks—ever since his grandmother back in Iowa had one installed below her right collarbone. According to Mike, she read her doctor the riot act.

"What were you thinking? I missed an entire hunting season! You can't shoot a shotgun with this thing in the way!"

◆   ◆   ◆

Of course, even as we began the fight on the body-wide chemotherapy front, we couldn't neglect the second front. The leg dressing had to be changed three times a day at Sacred Heart, just as it had at Navy. The difference was that the staffing level at Navy was much higher than at the civilian hospital. Navy had a bunch of nurses and hospital corpsmen on each shift. The very competent nurses at Sacred Heart were stretched thin. To maintain the sterile field during one dressing change, the nurse looked into the hall and flagged down a passing secretary to come in and open a dressing package for her. The poor woman wasn't prepared for the large open wound. While I wouldn't look at it myself, I did watch the faces of the people who did. Nancy thought the poor woman was going to faint. She managed not to gasp, but her eyes got big and she finally squeaked, "That's a big hole you've got there."

The "wound nurse" at Sacred Heart fascinated me. She was a retired Navy nurse who specialized in wound care. She really wanted to examine my leg, but she was extremely busy and never did coordinate her schedule with my schedule. She ended up asking my nurse to take a couple of photographs during one of my dressing changes—and to save the dressings so she could examine them. During the photo shoot, Nancy handed her camera to the nurse as well. Even though we both avoided looking, we thought that later on we might want to see what my leg had looked like.

When we took the roll of film to our local K-Mart, they shipped it off to a processor who initially refused to print those two pictures. I guess someone thought they were too graphic or gruesome. I was livid! I wanted to go right back to the store and light into the manager. Fortunately, Nancy took charge and called the company and explained that while some people might consider those pictures gross, I thought they were cancer-free and beautiful. They printed them the next time.

Sacred Heart hospital in Pensacola regularly earns accolades for their quality service to patients and families. The purple scrub-clad people hustling through the halls are the most upbeat and friendly hospital staff I've ever seen. I'll always remember Sacred Heart as a friendly, hard-working place where the hospital food is actually still hot when the tray reaches your room.

5

Back at Navy, Back in the Navy

SITREP #5

9/20/01

Dear Family, Friends, Shipmates, Argonauts, and IHMCers,

OK, I'm on the run again—back to room 53 in the Naval Hospital Pensacola. The lovely Nurse Nancy is getting the pack-out and move to a new room drill down to a science.

Finished the first course of chemo. Kinda wiped out today. I guess it wasn't a smart idea to stay up most of the night drinking barium contrast cocktails on any empty stomach. That's the drill to prepare for a CT scan, which we did this morning to make sure everything's still clear (it is). They give you a liter of foul fluid to drink at midnight, then feed you another bucket of the stuff for breakfast. Yum!

Also had a bone scan yesterday, which came out clean as a whistle. So now we are fighting the microscopic cells that may still exist. The next priority is to take care of the leg wound.

More later. Thanks for the calls, cards, and e-mails (I had over 150 yesterday).

GO USA! Larry

Before I was transferred from Sacred Heart back to Navy, Dr. Tan ordered some tests to check for any evidence of metastasized tumors anywhere else in my body. That is the usual course of Merkle cell. What starts out as an area of skin tumors very quickly spreads to other places in the body—places where it often kills. Fortunately, both the CT scan and the bone scan showed no evidence of cancer. If there is one good thing about an aggressive cancer like mine, it is that once you beat it the first time, you aren't sitting in remission limbo for too long. Recurrences show up quickly if they're coming. Dr. Tan told us that if you're clear of Merkle cell for two years, it almost assuredly isn't coming back.

◆   ◆   ◆

When I wrote SITREP #5 on September 20th, it was Day Four on the chemo calendar. Each new cycle began with three consecutive days of treatment. Looking back, I can't believe I got out of bed and got on the computer on Day Four. In future cycles, Day Four would mean only suffering. The first time around, I attributed my weariness and aching stomach to the preparations for the CT scan. While being unable to sleep most of the night and forcing down more than half a gallon of barium tracer certainly didn't help, the hung over feeling always came on Day Four, no matter what I ate or how I slept.

Chemotherapy introduced me to a level of fatigue I didn't know existed. I knew physical tiredness. I remember two-a-day football practice tiredness, 11 straight hours bailing hay tiredness, or four ballgames on Sunday with a five-hour drive home tiredness. After one particularly long and strenuous period at sea, I was so beat after thirty consecutive 18-hour days that I hit my rack as soon as we tied up in port. When I finally awoke, my clock said 6:30. The problem was that I honestly couldn't figure out if it was 6:30 in the morning or 6:30 in the evening! I had to go topside and check the sun.

But before chemo, I didn't know what it was like to be "Martha Stewart tired." Personally, I really don't care for Ms. Stewart's hugely successful television show. But during one of the few periods in which I was awake on that first Day Four, I found myself sitting up in my hospital bed when it came on my TV. The remote control was lying next to my left hip. Nevertheless, I watched the whole show because I couldn't summon the energy to change the channel. Now that's tired! Still, it was wonderful to be back with all our friends on 4 West at Navy.

SITREP #6

9/21/01

Dear Family, Friends, Shipmates, Classmates, Argonauts, and IHMCers,

A fine Navy day today for Nancy and me. First of all, I recovered from the first round of chemo treatments that had me asleep for about 20 hours yesterday. Stomach, energy, and appetite back to normal today.

Secondly, we found out that the Navy accepted my request to be returned to active duty for the duration of treatment. Being back on active duty simplifies the paperwork as far as paying for treatment. That's a relief! Nancy says that now that I'm back on active duty, I need a haircut. On the other hand—the chemo will take care of that soon enough!

The plan of attack calls for surgery this Monday to trim another few millimeters off the top edge of the shark bite and then close the wound with a skin graft. That may open up the possibility of getting out of the hospital a few days afterward. Yippee!

GO USA! Larry

Boy, was I stupid! Even though I knew I had cancer as the end of August approached, I suspect I was deep in denial about its potential severity. The inch-long cut at the biopsy site refused to heal, but I didn't worry. I thought it would make it simpler for Dr. Schneider to go back in and clean up any remaining cancerous tissue. I considered asking the Navy if having cancer would affect my official retirement date of September 1st. However, I was enjoying my new job so much that I didn't want to complicate matters. I let it slide. So, as far as the Navy bureaucracy was concerned, I became "USN Retired" as scheduled.

September 1st was Saturday of Labor Day weekend. When I returned to work the following Tuesday I should have taken a day to straighten out my remaining Navy paperwork—gotten a retired identification card, changed life insurance, and chosen our retiree medical treatment plan. Considering my medical situation, I cannot believe I didn't put those things at the top of my Do Points list. I'm sure I was denying the truth. I had convinced myself I'd have a simple surgery and leave the hospital the next day and live happily ever after. I promised myself to take care of the paperwork as soon as I got out of the hospital.

Besides, I had a big UWF research contract to get in place before I took off. I worked straight through Friday afternoon and got all parties to agree. I told everybody I'd be out a few days and had a great time with family and friends over the weekend.

While I screwed up and left myself in paperwork limbo, we could have eventually gotten that all straightened out...I think! The real question was whether or not I was truly qualified to retire. My mandatory retirement physical had been completed in March—about the time I first noticed the lump on my leg. The doctor didn't notice it then, and I didn't mention it. Now the results of that physical were obviously overtaken by events. All of us in Pensacola agreed that there was no way I should have retired in the middle of treatment.

Pam Long is the Active Duty Case Manager at the Naval Hospital in Pensacola. She is a bulldog when it comes to paperwork, and a terrific person to have on your side. She started working with Captain Phil Renaud, my good friend who was the METOC Officer detailer in the Bureau of Personnel in Memphis at the time. With the help of Phil's assistant, Brian Brown, they came up with a plan to fix the paperwork nightmare I had created.

Since the retirement paperwork had already been processed, the only way to fix the situation was for me to petition the Board of Correction of Naval Records. To my knowledge, the BCNR had never completed any petition action in less than two weeks. Using the medical information Pam gathered and a letter from Dr. Schneider, Phil and Brian drafted a letter to the Bureau for my signature. They faxed it to Pensacola. I signed it and Pam faxed it back to Memphis just before I left Navy for Sacred Heart. Phil forwarded it to the BCNR in Washington. He didn't just forward it. He greased the skids so well that two days later the BCNR signed out a finding letter that corrected my naval record to show that I was "not released from active duty on 31 August 2001 or transferred to the Retired List on 1 September 2001."

For 25 years I told people "the Navy takes care of its own." I'm living proof.

6

Closure

At Navy, we were back among friends. In nearly three weeks on the ward, Nancy and I made friends with all the nurses and corpsmen in the four watch sections. We knew the cafeteria workers, the nighttime pharmacist, the physical therapy staff, and the custodians. The aftermath of the terrorist attacks seemed to draw the whole hospital together. Everyone (except those of us who were inpatients) had to deal with greatly increased security measures in their comings and goings. Identification was checked at several points. Cars, purses, and packages were inspected. The corpsmen drew additional duty to augment the security staff. Patriotism was a common and welcome new subject. As in much of the country, you couldn't find a flag to buy in Pensacola. Friends sent us several and Nancy picked up some small ones from home. She decorated my room and handed out the extras to the hospital staff.

As the senior officer inpatient on the ward, I was treated royally. The charge nurse made up a "Captain's Quarters" sign for the door. Since the hospital was unusually un-crowded during that time, they let me stay in the big room with four beds. At one point, they offered to move me to a private room, but I wanted to stay in the room with the two phone lines. I used one for the computer and kept the other open for incoming calls. I used one of the other beds for all the books and magazines people sent. I figured I had one corner of the room for my bedroom, another for an office, a third for my library, while the fourth was my "guest room." I was perfectly willing to entertain a roommate, but the patient load never got to that point.

◆   ◆   ◆

On the Saturday after I returned from Sacred Heart to the Navy Hospital, I decided it was time to take a real shower. For the ten days up until then I had been trying to stay reasonably clean and fresh using sponge baths, "rinseless shampoo" and a washcloth at the small sink. It was less than satisfactory, especially when I had to spend so much time each day sitting and sleeping on the same set of sheets.

The corpsman on duty wrapped my lower leg in a plastic bag and taped it to keep the dressing dry. Then he brought me an extra plastic stool. I crutched my way into the bathroom, arranged my towel and toiletries in the sink, and got out of my gym shorts and hospital gown. Since I still couldn't put any weight on the injured leg, I did a one-legged hop up onto the edge of the shower stall. This was an accomplishment for me, since I have never been known for my leaping ability—even when I had two much younger legs. As a basketball player, I got my rebounds with long arms and good position, not by out-jumping my opponents. I put my soap and shampoo on the shelf and hopped around to sit on one plastic stool with my right leg sticking out around the shower curtain and propped on the other.

I looked up at the showerhead and realized that if I turned on the water from that position, I would be directly under the first blast of cold water. I struggled back to my foot, hopped back up onto the edge of the stall, and turned on the water to warm it up to a comfortable temperature. I don't know how long it had been since the last time someone took a shower in that bathroom, but the showerhead sprayed water in every direction. I reached for the sliding pin valve above the showerhead to shut down the water so I could try to adjust the spray. When I pushed on the button, the pin slid all the way through the valve and fell onto the floor of the shower. Now water was spraying directly over the curtain, out of the shower, and all over the bathroom floor. I finally got the water turned off and the pin back in the valve.

The corpsman heard me vent my frustrations with the condition of my plumbing. He yelled through the door, "You all right in there, sir?"

"Yeah, but can you find me a dry towel and a dry gown?"

I figured that everything was already soaked, so I might as well go ahead with the hot shower, wash my hair, and let the water spray where it would. A mop and bucket arrived with the dry towels. An hour later a maintenance man showed up with a new showerhead. The Saturday shower felt so good, I tested the new plumbing with another one on Sunday.

◆   ◆   ◆

Pensacola is not a Navy teaching hospital, but they still have a large number of young people who are in their first operational tour of duty. My case made for a good training opportunity. The staff of junior officer nurses and enlisted corpsmen was a pretty good mix of experience and youth. About half the nurses had worked their way up through the enlisted ranks before entering a commissioning program. These "mustang" officers were fun. One night shift lieutenant made sure her sailors brought me a Wendy's Frosty whenever they went on their food run. Many of these older nurses had spent their whole Navy career in medicine, having been hospital corpsmen during their enlisted service. But one ensign had spent her earlier active duty time as a parachute rigger and helicopter crewman. Ensign Cortez is cool. The first time she observed my leg without the bandages, she licked her lips and did a spot-on Hannibal Lecter impersonation.

The nurses allowed the young corpsmen to take turns changing my dressing for training and qualification. We had the dressing change procedure down to a science. The first item on the checklist was pain prevention. Twenty to thirty minutes in advance, the staff would stop by my room and tell me to hit the pain killer button. While I was attached to an IV, I had control of the morphine-based drugs. The supply was locked inside a box on Osama the IV stand, and I pressed a button to administer a dose. Since it was a strong narcotic, I tried not to use it very often—but I always made an exception at dressing change time. After I was finally detached from the IV, they brought me a couple of strong Percocet tablets half an hour before each change.

When dressing change time came, a nurse and corpsman would march in and gather up all their supplies. Most of the young folks had never seen a surgical wound like mine. As the word spread, the crowd of spectators grew. I should have sold tickets. The hole in my leg was apparently a big attraction for medical types. The nurses held impromptu anatomy classes. While they studied the inside of my leg, I would wiggle my toes. That usually brought a reaction.

"Whoa! Cool! Do that again, Captain!"

The more experienced folks also used me as a chance to teach bedside manner. It is important that corpsmen learn to control their own reaction to wounds and injuries. It is hard to keep the patient calm if the medic is upset. One very young corpsman took her first look at my wound and cringed.

"Is that a bone?"

Ensign Cortez snapped at her, "You can go stand in the passageway!"

SITREP #7

9/25/01

Dear Family, Friends, Shipmates, Classmates, Argonauts, and IHMCers,

I visited my friends in the Operating and Recovery Rooms again yesterday. We've been making it a weekly party. "If it's Monday, it must be surgery."

This week they did a skin graft to close the leg wound. The good news is that there are no more dressing changes! The bad news is that I'm on bed rest for a few days to make sure the graft isn't disturbed before it takes firm hold. The site is immobilized with a splint and all wrapped up in ace bandages. But believe me, bed confinement is enough to start wearing on a person's sunny disposition.

The donor site was from the top of my left thigh. It feels like I did a headfirst slide across a coral reef. As I told Lindsay, if you're a ballplayer—just imagine the worst sliding strawberry you've ever had. Ah well—pain is temporary.

If all goes well, the wraps and dressings will come off on Friday or Saturday. Maybe I can get out of here not long after that! The weather in Pensacola is perfect this week, and I'm staring out a window instead of going to the beach or watching a ball game. (Don't worry, I'll cover up and use good sunscreen. I strongly recommend you do the same!)

Nancy and I greatly appreciate the wonderful outpouring of support from all our great friends. She's been a tower of strength—putting up with my demands and running all the errands. Between Nanc and all the great folks at NAVHOSP Pensacola, I'm spoiled rotten.

GO USA! Larry

For the third week in a row I had surgery on my schedule for Monday. Dr. Schneider removed a few more millimeters from the upper edge of the wound, where the pathologists had identified microscopic cancer cells after the first surgery. Even though Mike trusted that chemo would get rid of them, as a surgeon, he preferred to completely wipe out the enemy on his front. I must admit that it was reassuring to have a clean margin all around the original tumor site. Provided the skin graft worked, I would be mobile by the end of the week.

After the skin graft the painful dressing changes on the lower right leg were history. But the agony of the dressing changes on the donor site on the left thigh more than made up for them. As gentle as the nurse tried to be, I know I used some words that I thought I had forgotten. But as the raw skin began to heal after a few days, Mike came up with a great solution. Using an amazing artificial skin stuff called tegaderm, he crafted a plastic patch over my thigh. He glued the edges down to my leg. The result was a breathable but waterproof protective shield. It could stay on my leg until the donor site was pretty much healed. I was finished with the painful dressing changes. Now, I do believe that pain is temporary, and it isn't necessarily bad for you. Nevertheless, I also believe it should be avoided whenever possible!

SITREP #8

9/28/01

Dear Family, Friends, Shipmates, Classmates, Argonauts, and IHMCers,

Hallelujah, I'm getting out of the hospital tomorrow (Saturday)! The bed rest was irritating—literally and figuratively—but the end result was good. The skin graft turned out great, and the donor site is beginning to heal. The IV is unplugged (so I don't have to deal with Osama the IV stand until the next chemo session). The tissue sample the surgeon took from the top edge of the "shark bite" (what's a few millimeters between friends, anyway?) was cancer-free, so we now know that we have a clean margin all around the original site.

I still can't put any weight on my right foot, and I have to keep it elevated most of the time. The right ankle and left thigh are pretty raw as new skin grows in both places. But I will finally be able to experience this week's great weather in the Florida Panhandle. Actually, we'll miss all the great people here at the Pensacola Naval Hospital. They've become great friends over the last three weeks.

We will be offline for a few days, until we can get a phone line connected in my apartment. I had been using a cell phone only, but will now need a regular line to use for the computer.

GO USA! Larry

7

God Bless America and Let's Play Ball!

SITREP #9

10/1/01

Dear Family, Friends, Shipmates, Classmates, Argonauts, and IHMCers,

Headquarters for the anti-cancer campaign have shifted from the Naval Hospital in Pensacola to my "temporary" furnished apartment in Pensacola. I rented this place in July with the intent of staying just a month or two until we were able to sell our house in LA and buy in FL. It's an old Sheraton that was converted to condos years ago. Our "penthouse" is 625 square feet—1 bedroom, 2 baths. I never expected to spend so much time in it!

We left the hospital Saturday and went straight to UWF, where the Argonauts were hosting a fall softball tournament. I can't think of a better incentive to get going! I wore my brand new "UWF Softball" t-shirt that Lindsay gave me. It was great to see her, Coach Cyr, all the Argos, plus other old softball friends. The Spring Hill College Badgers were in the tournament, and they have a number of players we know from Louisiana. The weather was ideal, so we stayed for about three hours.

Once again, I see unusual similarities between my personal situation and our world war on terrorism. While I have the utmost confidence in the commanders, the weapons, the troops, the plan of action, and ultimate victory, I question whether I have sufficient patience to put up with all the small inconveniences along the way.

The expected hair loss is one example. I have no problem with losing my hair (there isn't much where it's supposed to be anyway). I had Nancy break out the clippers last night and cut it all to an inch or shorter. It doesn't look bad! And I have this fond hope that at the end of the chemo, the follicles that have been dormant for years will magically reawaken. However, the day-to-day process is very irritating. Even though I don't have a lot on my head, the rest of my body is very long and pretty hairy. In my case, the loss started in places other than my head. I wake up in the morning in sheets full of hairs that have lost the good fight. Nancy says she is glad I'm shedding here, rather than in the house she's trying to sell in LA. Back at USNA, we dared other mids to try something by telling them, "You don't have a hair on your _ _ _ if you don't!" Well, now I can say, "Yep, you're right."

Immobility is another challenge to my patience. I don't mind being on crutches. Even being "non-weight bearing" (which makes you much slower than "partial weight bearing") is OK. Crutching around is the kind of physical challenge I enjoy. The thing that keeps me confined is the swelling in my foot. My size 13EE left foot looks small compared to the ballooned-up right foot. I must keep it elevated all the time to allow gravity to help. That means I spend way too much time sitting on my butt...and it hurts.

OK, enough of the whining. It's good to be back on the e-mail. Thank you for your continued prayers. Please add "patience" to the list—for me and for our country.

GO USA! Larry

I am a fastpitch softball fan. "Fan," of course, is short for "fanatic." Nancy feels I step back and forth across the fanatic line pretty often. Throughout my treatment and recovery I kept my sights on the 2002 season. I told the medical and physical therapy team that our goal was to have me umpiring again by the time summer ball started. I made reservations for the Argonauts' trip to the early March Leadoff Classic in Dallas. To those who know me well, it's no surprise that the first place I wanted to go upon getting discharged from the hospital was to a softball game.

My dad is a big baseball fan. My earliest memory in life is of our backyard in Smithsburg. I'm two—maybe three years old. Dad is trying to toss a rubber ball so that it hits the little wooden bat I swing wildly. (Whiffle balls and yellow plastic bats are still a few years away.) When he succeeds, I'm the happiest little boy in the world. Dad was a great player in his younger days. The talent skipped a generation in my particular branch of the family. I was better at football and basketball than baseball. But I definitely inherited Dad's love of the game.

Through the various stops of my Navy career, I organized and coached my command's slowpitch softball teams. Naturally, I volunteered to help coach T-ball as soon as Jim was old enough to play. (I also coached both kids' soccer teams for a couple of years, but once they were 8 or 9 years old, the players knew more than I did—and could beat me in the dribble relays.) When we were stationed in Italy, Jim and Lindsay played T-Ball on the same team. There were only enough kids for two teams. They played against the same opponent each week. My job on the Sixth Fleet staff kept me at sea so much that I didn't get to see them play very often. But we would take our gloves out and play catch whenever the flagship was in port.

Jim was a decent ballplayer, and one of the strongest hitters in Little League when we returned to Virginia for our next assignment. I still chuckle when I think of the night we drove home after I was the volunteer home plate umpire for one of his games. In the first three games of the season, he had reached base in every at bat, either by hit, walk, or error. In game four, I rung him up on a 3-2 pitch on the inside corner. Our conversation on the drive home went something like this:

"Dad, that pitch was inside!"

"It was too close to take!"

"It was inside!"

"It was close enough!"

We repeated the same general conversation several times before his next game. But Jim's team learned that if I was umpiring, you better hadn't get in the batter's box looking for a walk. They ended the season with the best batting average in the league—and won the championship.

Jim's other interests overtook sports when he reached high school. He became an Eagle Scout and won the Louisiana State Championship in the Duet Acting category of speech and debate. He enjoys acting, and he is a fine public speaker. He was chosen to give the graduation address for the FHS Class of 1999. He can still pound a golf ball, but neither of us is ever quite sure in what direction it's going to go.

◆   ◆   ◆

My beautiful baby daughter, though, grew up with both the talent and desire to excel in softball. My love of baseball quickly transferred to its much faster-paced cousin, women's fastpitch softball. I still enjoy baseball, but I don't drive 700 miles to go to baseball tournaments.

When she began playing, Lindsay was a star in our recreational league in Fairfax County, Virginia. I coached her team, assisted with our league All-Star team, became an ASA-certified umpire, and did most of the field maintenance. Nancy threatened to have my mail forwarded to the SYA field complex. I reasoned that she at least knew where to find me, and it wasn't in a bar.

At the urging of an Air Force officer named Bob Mathis, our little recreation association decided to form a "select" team to take part in 14-and-under fastpitch tournaments in the Washington, DC area. I was one of Bob's assistant coaches. He didn't even have a daughter on the team. He just loved the sport, and had some experience with travel ball.

We took a dozen of our local girls and went out to take on the best competition in the area. Rec league all-star teams are at a big disadvantage in travel ball. True travel ball teams recruit the best players from a wide area, and practice at least nine months a year. Still, we had some talented young ladies who worked hard. We were proud of how they played, even when traveling teams who came in from Oklahoma or Tennessee beat up on us. At least four girls from that Southwestern Fairfax County Youth Association team went on to play college softball. I'm still mighty proud of the Crusaders.

My next tour of duty took us to Stennis Space Center in Mississippi. We quickly decided that we would buy a house in Louisiana's St. Tammany Parish, where the public schools are pretty good and the softball was improving rapidly. A few months before we began our serious house hunting, I visited all the high schools in the parish. I think I really confused them when I asked to talk to the guidance counselor and the softball coach.

Shortly after we moved south, we contacted the local pitching expert, Bruce Desporte. He took Lindsay as a student, and we began a long-lasting friendship. Bruce's daughter Allison, (also known as Splinters) is a fine outfielder at the University of West Alabama, one of UWF's opponents in the Gulf South Conference. Whenever the Argonauts take on the UWA Tigers, Bruce and I get together to drink a beer or two and tell lies.

A new travel ball team was forming in the western St. Tammany area in the fall of 1995. Coach Becky Holliday was pleased to see an experienced left-handed pitcher show up for try-outs. High Voltage quickly established a reputation as one of the top organizations in the state. Through Lindsay's six years, we were never quite able to take the state championship, but we regularly finished among the top three teams in Louisiana. A number of former Volts are now playing college softball, and there are a number of talented players still working their way through the organization's different age groups.

I volunteered to be the High Voltage Sports Information Director, and soon added the Treasurer duties to my resume. We built our own practice field on a former Christmas tree farm, and erected a batting cage in the backyard of the Volt president, Francis Motichek. Francis and his wife Jobet kept the organization running through its first six years. As our daughters moved on to college, we turned over the Volts to younger families. It takes an amazing amount of work to organize and equip as many as four teams to play serious travel softball. The friends we made through High Voltage are some of the finest people you could ever want to meet. I wrote this poem for our organizational newsletter. It was published in *FastPitch World* magazine and I've since seen it copied on nearly two dozen softball websites, and it's even morphed into a baseball version.

THEN I BECAME A SOFTBALL DAD

I used to have a regular life. (Actually, many of my friends say that sentence should say, "I used to have a <u>life</u>", period.) It doesn't seem that long ago. Then I became a Softball Dad.

My lawn used to be like a carpet. It was green, mowed, trimmed, fertilized, and watered. Any weeds that dared to show their leaves were pulled out by their roots. Now I have two big bare spots forty feet apart. I like the bare spots, because they are the only places that the weeds and crab grass aren't threatening to take over.

My car used to draw admiring looks and comments. It was clean and waxed and shined and Armor All'd. Now it only draws attention when it wins the "dirtiest car in the parking lot" prize.

My friends and I used to spend Monday mornings talking about five-iron shots, three-putts, and titanium shafts. Now I bore them to death with detailed play-by-play descriptions of five or six low-scoring ball games. Somehow, they just don't understand the drama of a 2-0 game.

I used to think anything over $40 was an exorbitant price for a ball bat. Now the contents of my daughter's equipment bag are worth more than my entire travel bag—including clothes, watch, and laptop computer.

I used to have a great wife. Still do, Thank God. But that's a tribute to her patience and good humor. We used to sit and talk for hours. We still do—to keep the driver awake when we're headed home in the wee hours of Monday morning. We used to wonder what the kids would do when they grew up. Now she wants to know what I'm going to do <u>IF</u> I ever grow up.

My summer casual wardrobe used to be made up of color-coordinated polo shirts, cool cottons in bright colors, and the occasional "aloha" shirt. Now I have a closet full of T-shirts in royal blue. Those that don't have our team name on the front have a cute saying on the back, like "If You Follow Me Long Enough, You'll End Up at a Ballfield."

> I used to glue myself to the sofa and watch the NCAA basketball tournament, the Masters, and the NBA playoffs from opening ceremony through network sign off. Now, I catch the highlights on Sportscenter.
>
> I used to have sympathy for umpires.
>
> I used to think boys were tough.
>
> I used to think a double-header was a long day at the ball field. Now we're just getting warmed up.
>
> We used to spend our summer vacation relaxing on the beach or visiting family. Now we hit the road with 40 of our closest friends.
>
> I used to think the ideal woman had brains and beauty. She still does, but now she better also be quick, courageous, and able to bunt a good rise ball.
>
> I used to look for little restaurants that served seafood fresh off the boat. Now I'm a connoisseur of nachos and smoked sausages.
>
> I used to be concerned that I would fall into the trap of living my life through my daughter. Now I know that I'm privileged to live my life WITH my daughter.

Even if I do say so myself, Lindsay was the hardest working player on every one of her teams throughout her summer ball and high school ball years. She was usually the first one at practice, and the last to leave. She listened to her coaches and did whatever they instructed.

The hard work paid off in the 2000 season. She had been the number one pitcher for Fontainebleau High ever since her freshman year. In her junior year, she pitched nearly every game, batted clean up, and led the Bulldogs to the District co-championship. Against Ruston High School in the first round of playoffs, she struck out 12 and hit two home runs. In the Volt summer season she was 25-5, and led the team in home runs, runs batted in, slugging percentage, and walks.

As she began her senior year in the fall of 2000, she attracted some interest from college softball coaches. She said "No, thank you" to schools that weren't in the southeast. She likes playing in warm weather, and she likes having Dad at her games—almost as much as I like being there. By Christmas she had narrowed her choices down to UWF and two other schools. All three had very nice coaches, fine softball programs, and good academic reputations. After carefully weighing every factor we could think of, she picked West Florida.

Argonaut Coach Tami Cyr runs a terrific program on a limited budget. She doesn't have much scholarship money to spread around. One of the other schools combined softball and academic scholarships to offer Lindsay a full ride. While either of the other two schools would have cost us less out-of-pocket than UWF, we encouraged Lindsay to go where she really wanted to go. Tami was able to offer Lindsay a partial scholarship, which she verbally accepted in January. It was a proud day when she signed a National Letter of Intent at the opening of the April signing period.

Coach Cyr was wonderfully helpful through my cancer war. She always made sure Lindsay was OK and encouraged me to stay upbeat. *NEVER, NEVER, NEVER GIVE UP!* Right Tami?

◆   ◆   ◆

So, when I left the Navy hospital on September 29th, headed out in gorgeous Florida Panhandle fall sunshine to a softball tournament, I was a happy man. I figured out how to get myself and my crutches in and out of Nancy's minivan, and how to sit behind her and prop my foot on the front passenger seat.

We took a spot in the front row of the stands with my leg resting on a pillow on a stool. The Argonauts weren't playing in the game that was going on at the moment. Lindsay and Tami and a lot of the team members came over to say hello. That's when I bled all over the bleachers. The only problem with Doctor Mike's tegaderm patch was that it trapped all the blood and fluid that was still oozing from the skin donor site on my left thigh. With all the walking around on crutches, it had worked its way under the glued-down edge. Once it made it to the edge, about a pint of blood spilled on the concrete under the stands.

Lindsay had to get Vernita the trainer to come wrap my leg and tape it. I changed into a clean pair of gym shorts and we enjoyed the rest of the afternoon at the prettiest softball field in the Gulf South Conference.

8

Road Trip!

Dear Family, Friends, Classmates, Shipmates, Argonauts, and IHMCers,

Mobility is one of the principles of warfare. The ability to quickly move our forces where they had the most impact was a key in Desert Storm. It will also be crucial in the World War on Terrorism. That's why Secretaries Powell and Rumsfeld are visiting potential allies to insure we have the bases and overflight permissions we will need.

I doubt that mobility plays the same important role in the war on cancer (I don't think I can outrun it or hide from it), but Nancy and I are practicing mobility anyway. We have a week off between doctor appointments and my next chemotherapy session is now scheduled for October 17, 18, and 19. We decided to make a road trip to Mandeville to stay in more comfortable surroundings and visit friends. Nancy is even going to get to work a day or two at her part time job at the Magic Box. She misses all her toy store friends.

My personal mobility is improving, too. My surgeon said I could start testing the ankle, so I'm now putting some weight on it and stretching. Of course, that makes it hurt, but this is really a case where the old "no pain, no gain" saying is true. I figure the more I do now, the less I'll have to do in physical therapy later. It's a trade-off, though. At the same time, I'm trying to cut down on the heavy-duty pain pills. I have a good incentive. Once I'm managing the pain with Motrin, I can have a beer again. I feel like I've been at sea for a month—and the Abita Brewing Company probably wonders what happened to their Mandeville sales!

We'll be back in P'cola the middle of next week. As always, your thoughts, prayers, cards, and calls mean the world to me (especially the prayers). I've got to tell you about one get-well card. My "family" at the Naval Oceanographic Office sent a 3 x 5 card—three FEET by five FEET! It took me an hour to read all the nice words—one of the best hours I've had in months. Thanks y'all...you are the greatest!

Go USA! Larry

I never intended to spend much time in the apartment I rented in downtown Pensacola. When I signed the lease in mid-July, I hoped to only spend the workweek there for a month or two. We expected to sell our Louisiana house by early fall and move into our new home in western Florida. So the fact that the apartment was tiny, dark, and rather shabby didn't bother me. I didn't spend much time there. It was convenient to my office, and the TV and refrigerator worked.

Before surgery, Nancy had only spent a few nights in the apartment when she was in town on house-hunting trips. While I was hospitalized, she moved in. I was a bit worried about her, because the area is so empty at night. An interstate on-ramp, the Pensacola Civic Center, a cemetery, and the historic district of the city surrounded the condominium complex. It wasn't that it was unsafe. It was just lonely. I asked her to call me in my hospital room when she was safely "home" each night.

On the first Saturday night, she told me there were a lot of Pensacola police on the road as she got close to our place. As she got closer, she realized they were concentrated in our parking lot. Some of the other residents were with the police, checking people entering the lot to make sure they lived there. Seems the empty building next door had been rented out for an all night Rave Party. Shortly after she finally got to sleep, somebody pulled the fire alarm in our building. The ear-splitting alarm forced her outside into the same parking lot. It was a long night for Nurse Nancy.

During my three weeks in the hospital, Nancy made several overnight trips to Louisiana. Our home was on the market, but we continued to get our mail and bills there. About once a week she made the three-hour drive to pick up mail and check on the house. The trips gave her a welcome break from the apartment and the hospital routine.

We spent my first week out of the hospital cooped up in the apartment. I wasn't able to move around very much, so I monopolized the sofa. Nancy didn't have much to do. She didn't feel like house hunting because of the new level of uncertainty that had been injected into our lives. When it dawned on us that we had a whole week between medical appointments, we didn't have to twist each other's arms to get us on the road to our big house in Louisiana.

◆　　◆　　◆

In the 24 years of marriage before cancer we had evolved an easy workload-sharing agreement. When we traveled, I hauled the stuff to the car and packed it. Nancy did most of the driving, since we were usually in her minivan. When we reached our destination, I unpacked and hauled everything inside. But now, the whole workload fell on Nancy. The morning we left Pensacola, she got up, dressed, cooked breakfast for both of us, stripped the bed, packed our bags, hauled everything down to the parking lot, and packed the car. I managed to dress myself, and then sat on my butt until she told me it was time to get into the car. On the road, Nancy drove while I took a nap to recover from the strenuous exertion of getting into the car.

◆　　◆　　◆

My ankle still had dressings to change every day. During the skin graft, the surgeons used a dermatome (think of a sharp, sterile cheese slicer) to peel very thin strips of skin from the donor site. They formed them into a mesh, laid it over the granulation tissue, and stitched the edges. Mike said they would be happy with 70 percent coverage of healthy skin when the dressings came off. The skin would eventually grow to cover the remaining open areas. In my case they achieved more than 80 percent. But until it was completely healed, I still had to cover and protect it. Every morning I would remove the old dressing, shower, apply Minerin lotion, cover the area with four telfa pads, and wrap everything in a roll of gauze and an Ace bandage.

At my checkup before our road trip, Doctor Mike told me to start putting weight on my right foot. After four weeks, I really had to stretch the leg muscles and ligaments before I could even get the sole flat to the floor. I continued to use the crutches, but added more and more weight to the injured leg. It hurt, but not as much as I feared. Swelling was a bigger problem than pain.

Nearly half of the lymphatic circulation system around my ankle had been removed or interrupted. Mike explained that what was left was like a country road that had to take all of the cars and trucks detoured from a closed interstate highway. There was a route, but it couldn't handle the traffic volume. The removal of five lymph nodes from the groin complicated the problem. Mike was a little concerned that swelling of the whole leg would result. The more time I spent exercising the leg, the more the foot and lower leg swelled. Fortunately, the human body is pretty efficient in widening and building new roads to replace damaged ones. Over time, swelling became less of a problem. But for the first month, I had to spend almost all of my time with my foot elevated.

Once I started testing my leg, I made surprising progress. After a day of adding more and more weight, I put away the crutches. Nancy came home from a day at the Magic Box toy store to find me hobbling along on Jim's Boy Scout walking stick. Before the weekend was over, I put away the cane and shuffled along without artificial support. It felt great! Perhaps the best part was taking a shower standing up instead of sitting on a plastic stool.

At the same time that I was increasing my mobility, I was trying to wean myself from the heavy-duty painkillers. It was a classic trade-off. The more I worked on strength and flexibility, the more pain I felt. Still, I wanted to stop the prescription medicines. I reduced my Percocet consumption from the allowed twelve per day to three or four. Then I went to only over-the-counter ibuprofen. The pain in my ankle wasn't too bad, but during the weeks on powerful painkillers I had forgotten how much my arthritic knees always ached!

Like most of America, I had made a habit of living without enough sleep. Before cancer, I existed on six to seven hours rest per night. I knew it wasn't enough, but I was always too busy to make sleep a priority. In the wake of surgery and the first round of chemotherapy, I found to my surprise that I could sleep for ten to twelve hours at night—and still need a nap in the afternoon! I didn't appreciate how much energy the body required to heal. I usually felt pretty good from the time I got up in the morning until dinner. But I ran out of gas very quickly in the evening.

◆   ◆   ◆

The best part about going back to Louisiana was getting together with our friends. Nancy really missed all her coworkers and customers at the Magic Box. In fact, I received cards from several of her regular customers I didn't even know. They wanted me to get well so that Nancy could return to selling them toys! She worked two days during this trip home, and it was rejuvenating for her.

We also saw neighbors, softball friends, and some of the Navy family we knew so well. The Naval Oceanographic Office at Stennis Space Center, MS is the largest organization in the Navy's meteorology-oceanography business. "NAVO" has about a thousand dedicated employees. Most of them are civilian scientists and engineers. In fact, the largest concentration of professional oceanographers in the world is at Stennis! It's my personal opinion that being commanding officer of NAVO is the best job in the Navy. That was my job from 1997 until 2000. The NAVO people are like family to me. They sent me a steady stream of cards and e-mails through the entire duration of the war. Pat Smith made it his personal responsibility to call me every other week on his day off, just to ask how I was doing and shoot the bull for a few minutes.

We were in Louisiana over Columbus Day weekend, and our Navy friends wanted to entertain us. Nancy explained that I was pretty lousy company in the evening, so they invited us for lunch. On Sunday we went to the Mississippi Coast for lunch and a Saints TV football party at the NAVO Executive Officer's house. On Monday we went around the corner in Mandeville to the Commanding Officer's house for another nice luncheon with great friends.

9

OK, But Why Me?

SITREP #11

10/12/01

Dear Family, Friends, Shipmates, Classmates, Argonauts, and IHMCers,

Today's Pensacola News Journal quotes the President, "We've got them on the run." I've always felt that a nice, clear bomb damage assessment (BDA) photo of a former terrorist camp does the heart good!

I'm not exactly "on the run," but I did walk in to my doctor's appointment this morning carrying my crutches. Y'all thought I was a slow runner before—you ought to see me amble along now! The skin-grafted "shark bite" is healing nicely. Even Nurse Nancy checked it out this morning. She says it's not gruesome anymore (but that it's still rather ugly). Kids will definitely believe that a shark took a piece! Adults, too, for that matter. There's a lot of healing to do before I can go barefoot on the beach. I'm anxious to start Physical Therapy.

The skin donor site is nicely recovered, although the replacement skin seems to come in a different color. My thigh looks like a test patch for a new Crayola shade. It's one of those pink, purple, and white combinations that women instinctively know the name of (and men will always call "kinda pinkish-purple").

After getting welcome positive news from Dr. Mike, we stopped by Physical Therapy to turn in the crutches. Then we visited our friends (the nurses, staff, and corpsmen) on 4 West. On the way out, we went to the Mail Room. I'm glad we did, because there were forty cards and four packages waiting for me! (Somehow, they never got a forwarding address.) So those of you who mailed things to me in the hospital last month—THANKS!

Three of the packages contained books that I look forward to reading. That's one of the positives of this ordeal—I get to read books I've wanted to read for ages. The fourth package contained a little stuffed kangaroo with a faded backpack, a wrinkled blue shirt, and chain-link fence marks on his ears. (The High Voltage softball players know exactly what I'm talking about. I'll try to be worthy. Thanks, Roo!)

Chemo session number two is next Wednesday, Thursday, and Friday. It's doing a number on my hair. I have faith it's also got the cancer "on the run."

GO USA! Larry

From the day the wraps came off the skin graft, I was impatient to have the ankle wound fully closed. I had no idea it would take as long as it did. Eventually I got pretty good at the dressing-change routine. Every day before my shower I would throw away the old gauze wraps and telfa pads. After showering I rubbed in moisturizing lotion and re-dressed the wound. It actually got to be a comforting part of my routine.

Still, I was anxious to have it healed. We asked Doctor Mike when the skin would grow over the remaining holes. He patiently explained that it normally takes only a couple of weeks…if you aren't undergoing chemotherapy at the time! But the microscopic soldiers my body needed to close the wound on the ankle front were being sacrificed on the chemotherapy front. So my toiletry kit contained Kerlix gauze rolls and Ace bandages for many months. It was another chance for me to practice patience. Somehow, even with all the practice, I never became noticeably more patient.

◆　　◆　　◆

The seabag full of mail we picked up at the hospital mailroom was a huge spirit-lifter. There were cards from friends all over the world. Personally, I like the funny ones. I guess most people think there isn't anything humorous about cancer. And they are certainly right about that. So I can understand why people are reluctant to send funny get well cards to a cancer patient. That made me treasure the rare humorous ones even more. After all, life is chock full of really funny situations. You have to hone your sense of humor and develop your ability to spot the potential belly laughs. Then you have to take time out to enjoy them. Laughter is great medicine.

My favorite thing out of everything in the mailbag was the stuffed toy kangaroo. Ronette Wright is one of the great young ladies who played softball for High Voltage. She's a speedy outfielder from Ponchatoula, LA. The team always called her "Roo." During the 2000 season she bought a small version of Winnie the Pooh's Roo from the Disney Store the girls visited on one of our trips.

"T'Roo"—which is Cajun for Petite Roo, or Little Roo—went to every Volt game from that point on. Ronette hung him from the chain link fence near our dugout. When she sent him to me, she told me he had seen a lot of victories, and was ready to cheer me on to one more. He sat with me in my recliner when I went to chemotherapy. The nurses and even the other patients looked forward to T'Roo's trips to the treatment room. Even six months later, when I returned for my quarterly check up, the nurse asked me how my mascot was doing.

◆   ◆   ◆

The books were also a welcome treat. Reading has always been one of my favorite pastimes. It seems like it always takes me a quite a while to get through each book. Partly, it's because I don't concentrate on only one book until I finish it. At any point in time, I am usually in the middle of two or three books and a couple of magazines. But mostly, it's because I don't devote enough time to pleasure reading. Like sleep, it was one of the things I never put high enough on my priority list before cancer. Convalescence gave me the time to catch up. I read cancer books. I read inspirational books. I read history, spy novels, magazines, and Harry Potter. I even did a little patient-level research on Merkle cell carcinoma and cancer in general.

Not surprisingly, it didn't take me long to get over my head in the cancer journals. The science of oncology is one of the most exciting areas of research for some of the smartest people in the country and the world. I tried to build my own mental model to help me better understand cancer. My version is about as elementary as they come. If it were to answer one of his essay questions, my high school biology teacher would probably give me about half credit. Cancer researchers, like my classmate and good friend, Carl June, probably shudder when they read it. But my "Idiot's Guide to Cancer Cells" helped me understand what might have happened to me.

◆   ◆   ◆

The cells in our body reproduce by mitosis, or cell division. That is how we grow new cells to build muscle and tissue and to replace old cells. Within the estimated sixty trillion cells in each of our human bodies, there are billions of cell divisions happening every day. A very small percentage of these cell divisions don't proceed normally. Damage to the DNA results in imperfect copies. These defective copies usually are unable to reproduce themselves. But a very small percentage of the defects reproduce rapidly. Fast-growing abnormal cells form malignant tumors—cancer. If our immune system is strong, it will detect these malignancies, target them, and wipe them out before they can grow out of control.

Smoking, excess sun, exposure to carcinogens, exposure to radiation, heredity, or poor diet can lead to a greater number of errors in mitosis, an increased occurrence of abnormal cell divisions—and a greater chance of cancer. Similarly, we can weaken our own immune systems by not feeding ourselves a healthy diet, by not getting enough sleep, or by lack of exercise. Living with too much stress also plays havoc with the immune system.

◆   ◆   ◆

From the day of my diagnosis, I couldn't understand why cancer would attack me. I went through all five stages of grief—denial, anger, bargaining, depression, and finally—acceptance. It's too bad you don't get to march through the grieving process in a nice, neat, predictable order. It would be easier if you could set up a checklist and just go down the stages and mark them off. "OK, I'm done with the anger part. Let's go on to bargaining." In real life you bounce back and forth through the first four stages until you eventually reach an acceptance of your loss. There's no timeline—and no guarantee that you have the anger and depression behind you for good. Just when you think you've got them all licked, they sneak back in on you in a weak moment.

I was angry that I had cancer. I was especially angry because I had worked so hard to live the kind of healthy lifestyle that would supposedly keep me free of disease. For my entire adult life I had exercised, maintained a healthy weight, eaten well, and generally taken care of myself. Nancy is a great cook. She majored in Home Economics at Hood College. (That politically incorrect major has sadly disappeared from the curriculum. Too bad.) We eat a well-balanced diet that is pretty low in fried foods and red meat and high in pasta, chicken, and fresh fruits and vegetables. Blueberries, one of the best anti-cancer foods of all, are my favorite fruit. I was even ahead of my time in alcohol consumption. I made it a habit to drink a daily beer or two or a glass of red wine many years before scientists proved that they were actually healthy.

Before cancer, I exercised five or six days a week. I rarely pushed myself very hard, but I would combine weight lifting with stretching, walking, bicycling, stair climbing, and the aerobic machines in the Wellness Center. When running errands I looked for the chance to burn a few extra calories. I took the stairs instead of the elevator. I parked in the first open space in supermarket parking lot, rather than driving around searching for one near the door.

Back in the days when my knees hurt didn't hurt so much, jogging, racquetball, and basketball were staples of my exercise program. Now my aerobic work is limited to walking and elliptical trainers, which don't pound the joints. The knee damage dates to high school days, and has been aggravated by years of abuse in gyms and on ships. They finally wore out a few years ago. The orthopedic folks tell me that I'll some day be the proud owner of titanium knees. I think I'll delay as long as I can and give the artificial joint technology researchers more time to continue to improve the product.

With a family history of high blood pressure, I watch mine closely, and have for a long time. Years ago I bought an electronic BP and pulse device that I keep in my office desk. Every couple of years I take it with me on a visit to the clinic and have it calibrated. I monitor my cholesterol count regularly. I am fortunate that my total cholesterol is always below 170, with a great ratio of "good" to "bad."

More than anything else, I was proud that I maintained a healthy balance in my life. I took time off to enjoy my family, my hobbies, travel, and relaxation. I made it a point of pride to resist the Navy's workaholic tradition. Most U.S. Navy officers work unbelievably long hours. The Navy culture encourages its people to imitate and look up to those hard-working officers who get in to the office first and leave last. I've always figured that made perfect sense when you're at sea and don't have anything else to do anyway.

But I didn't see the necessity of working the same crazy hours when the ship was in port or I was assigned to shore duty. As an ensign stationed on my first ship, I decided that I would break the accepted tradition and leave the ship at a reasonable hour. Later in my career I would occasionally have a boss challenge my "short" working hours. My standard answer was, "I can't help it everyone else can't finish their work during normal hours."

So there I was—happy, healthy, balanced, and in good physical condition with a great positive outlook on life. Why did I have cancer? That question bugged me for weeks! My acceptance kept backsliding to anger.

Cheryl Shank is a cancer warrior friend who was one of my coaches during my cancer experience. Years ago she survived against pretty steep odds. Cheryl gave me one of the best books I read during my war. *The Cancer Conqueror* is out of print, but Cheryl got a copy from Amazon's used books section. When I read it, I finally began to see the light.

The author talks about how our lifestyle can make us more susceptible to cancer. As I said, I thought I was in great shape. I never smoked in my life (except for one horrible tasting cigar during a poker night in Naples). My diet isn't perfect, but it's pretty darn good. My weight is right. I definitely get too much sun, but I've been a faithful user of sunscreen for years. Then I got to the section about the impact of stress on our lives. The writer suggested to the cancer warrior in the story that she think back over the past two years and judge the impact of stress on her life.

At first glance, I thought that stress couldn't possibly be the problem. For thirty years I had dealt with one of the most stressful lifestyles imaginable. Navy families are routinely separated for months at a time. We move to new duty stations when we are just getting settled in the old ones. As we advance in our careers, we get new jobs or new bosses nearly every year. Heck, I even survived five years of Washington DC traffic. I thought I was immune to stress.

But I went through the exercise anyway, and was surprised at what I found. Beginning a year before I noticed the lump on my leg, I cataloged the stressors in my life, and was surprised at how a collection of apparently small and unrelated problems had accumulated so quickly.

◆   ◆   ◆

In March 2000, one year before I first noticed the lump, I judged my life to be nearly perfect. I was happily married to the love of my life. We had good jobs, a beautiful house, and great children. My Navy career was better than I had ever hoped. I was set to turn over the command of the Naval Oceanographic Office after an exceptional thirty months in the best job in the Navy. I had reached the Navy goal I had set years before—to make Captain and be a solid contender for promotion to Rear Admiral.

Jim was doing superbly in his sophomore year at Tulane University in New Orleans. He had terrific grades, a smart and sweet girlfriend, a role in the spring play, and a good summer job to return to in May. He was going to Tulane on a full-tuition Dean's Honors Scholarship. He augmented that with money from a Toyota Scholarship he won in high school and some more from Louisiana's TOPS program that encourages the state's high school graduates to stay at in-state colleges. Most of the money we had saved for his college fund was still in the bank for graduate school.

Lindsay was a junior in high school with a bunch of nice friends, honor roll grades, and a full schedule of extracurricular activities. She was also in the middle of an outstanding high school softball season in which she would earn the school's pitching, hitting, and Most Valuable Player awards. She was voted the Outstanding Player in one of Louisiana's better large-school softball districts. She was the St. Tammany Parish MVP and made Honorable Mention All State, even though the Bulldogs missed out on a trip to the state tournament.

Over the next twelve months, though, I experienced a series of stressful events in my life. Most of them were unrelated. Individually, they didn't seem too serious. We didn't have to live through the biggest life stressors, like divorce or the death of a loved one. But in retrospect, the collective weight of the stress accumulated quickly as each new event forced its way into our lives.

On Saint Patrick's Day 2000 we celebrated my outgoing Change of Command at NAVO. This ceremony is a normal milestone for a naval officer, and it was a fun celebration with a standing-room only crowd. Still, I was giving up the best job in the Navy to go to a new job as the admiral's Chief of Staff.

The Chief of Staff holds a position of respect and responsibility, but it just isn't as much fun as being the boss of a large organization. In command, I had been responsible for a thousand people, eight ships, and a yearly budget of $120 million of the taxpayer's hard-earned money. The responsibility of command is surely stressful by itself, but it was an invigorating kind of stress that made going to work everyday a pleasure. Running the admiral's staff was equally stressful, but just wasn't as much fun. ***Strike one***.

A month after I started my new job we had a crisis with the High Voltage 16-and-under team. The summer between a softball prospect's junior and senior years in high school is the key season for girls who desire to play the game in college. It is the chance to be seen by college coaches who are starting to make their recruiting plans for that graduating class.

One of our star players was in the same high school class as Lindsay. She won the district Outstanding Player award as a sophomore. Lindsay won it their junior season. Her parents decided, just before the summer season began, to desert our team for a chance to play for a more recognized organization in Baton Rouge. Girls often change teams from one year to the next, but the change is typically made in the fall. Once rosters are set, most people remain loyal to their team. Through this last minute betrayal, the team not only lost a terrific player, but I personally lost the friendship of her parents. Plus, we had to find a last-minute replacement for one of the superstar players on our roster. It kept me awake at night for a week. ***Strike two***.

In late May, the results of the admiral selection board were announced. I didn't know what to expect. The small community of Meteorology-Oceanography (METOC) specialists has just one flag officer job. As it is a 36-month assignment, we promote one of our officers to Rear Admiral only once every three years.

When he headed the METOC Command, Vice Admiral Paul Gaffney, made it his goal to have a handful of highly qualified officers for the selection board to consider. (Admiral Gaffney is a great friend and my personal mentor. He is so good that the Navy made an exception in his case. Rather than letting him retire after his three years in charge of the METOC Command, they promoted him to two stars as the Chief of Naval Research, and then to the three-star rank of Vice Admiral. He is the president of the National Defense University.) He believed that we have so many high quality officers that it would be a disservice to the country for him to single out one person to be his successor.

Admiral Gaffney was relieved in 1997 by Rear Admiral Ken Barbor, an old friend and my new boss. Admiral Barbor agreed with the Gaffney promotion concept, so my selection board had at least six outstanding officers from which to pick. I knew I had a good record, and friends kept telling Nancy that I was sure to be selected. I tried to tell her that the odds were against it, but I don't think the message got through.

The Navy promotion process is inherently fair and almost always results in wise choices. I told Admiral Barbor not to worry about the outcome. With the group they had to choose from, the selection board could not possibly make a mistake. But as fair as it is, the selection board process occasionally involves some degree of luck. If one of the officers being considered happened to work for one of the admirals sitting on the board, that officer has an advantage (provided the admiral liked his work, of course).

One of my Naval Academy classmates had twice worked for the senior officer on the selection board. He also had an outstanding record, and was named the new commander. As much as I tried to be prepared, it still hurt. It was the first time in our careers that the other five of us had failed to be chosen by a selection board. Nancy took it harder than I did. She really believed that I was the best (as each one of our wives surely believed). ***Strike three. One out. Next batter.***

Any parent who has gone through the college-choosing and application process knows that it can be a trying time. Throughout that summer and fall of 2000, Lindsay was trying to figure out where she would go to college. When your child is faced with a big decision, it is quite stressful for parents. Having gone through the process with Jim two years before, I knew it was hard. Lindsay's choice was complicated by the softball recruiting process. I wouldn't call her a "blue-chip" prospect, but she did receive some interest from a dozen different schools. Being recruited is exciting, but it definitely adds to the stress of choosing a school. After narrowing the list, we visited half a dozen fine universities and talked to some dedicated coaches. It wasn't easy.

Another softball dad sent me this story.

> A young softball star died tragically. When she reached the Pearly Gates, St. Peter told her that her short life had been a good one, and that she had earned the right to choose where she would spend eternity. First, she made an official visit to Hell. Satan took her to the most beautiful softball field she had ever seen. The grass of the outfield was green and soft and mowed like a fairway at Pebble Beach. The infield dirt was perfectly groomed. The players were dressed in the slickest new dazzle-cloth uniforms. The bat rack was filled with hot new Demarinis and brand-new balls overflowed from the carpeted locker room. The coach and the players were extremely nice to the girl. The weather was sunny and warm. They played a doubleheader, and then went out for a great steak dinner at a nice restaurant.
>
> The player returned to Heaven, where she was shown a nice fluffy cloud, a harp, a halo, and a new pair of wings. She agonized overnight before finally telling St. Peter that Heaven was very nice, but she really wanted to play softball. St. Peter said, "As you wish" and sent her back to Hell. She arrived to find the coach screaming

at a team of players dressed in rags and picking endless rocks off an ugly, scrubby field full of bare spots and holes. The bats were dented and the only ball was worn smooth and brown. It was as hot as Hades. She turned to Satan and said, "But yesterday everything was so nice!" The devil replied, "Ah yes. But yesterday you were being recruited. Today you're on the team."

Another strike.

While Lindsay was spending the summer weighing the pluses and minuses of different colleges, Nancy and I made the big decision to retire from the Navy in 2001. We had known the new admiral for many years, and I knew that our styles were very different. Working as his Chief of Staff would be difficult for me. It was time to move on to the next chapter of our lives. This decision led to several more questions. Where did we want to live? What did I want to do? Could I find a job doing what I wanted to do in the place where we wanted to be?

The Navy recognizes the stress that comes when our people reach the end of their active duty careers. They offer weeklong seminars to teach officers and senior enlisted people how to prepare for entry into the civilian job market. Since most military folks enter active duty right out of high school or college, we are unfamiliar with networking, interviewing, and negotiating contracts. Most of us need advice in choosing a business wardrobe. I attended two of these transition seminars and began networking in search of a good civilian job, preferably in the Florida Panhandle.

I was confident that I would land an interesting position in the real world. As a friend pointed out, all of the officers we had worked with throughout our careers and who had retired before us were working at post-Navy jobs. Nobody was on welfare. Still, for someone who last interviewed for a job flipping burgers at age 16, the whole job-hunting process was a stressful mystery. **Strike two.**

The fall of 2000 was hectic at work. I was responsible for the impending retirement dinner and ceremony for Ken Barbor and his wife, Leslie. I tried to balance that with helping coordinate the first few weeks of my classmate's life as the new admiral in Mississippi. ***Strike three. Two outs. Next hitter.***

Additionally, the staff moved from our old headquarters to a newly constructed building at the Stennis Space Center. I had to ensure all our files and phones and furniture were packed and unpacked without shutting down business. ***Strike one.*** These headaches came on top of the usual full schedule involved in running a worldwide command employing three thousand active duty and civilian personnel. ***Strike two.***

On top of everything else, an injury to Lindsay was easily the most stressful occurrence out of everything that happened during that stress-filled year. In the last tournament of the summer season she played the best softball of her life. In eight games at the ASA regional tournament in Oklahoma City we faced the best teams from Oklahoma, Arkansas, Louisiana, Mississippi, and western Tennessee. Lindsay batted .500 and beat the Oklahoma City L'il Saints in the last game she pitched. High Voltage finished third in the regional and earned a berth in the National Championship Tournament. Unfortunately, by that point in the season, we were out of money and ballplayers. The lobby of our hotel on Saturday night looked like a M.A.S.H. unit. The Volts finished an unbelievable season with a record of 51-10. On the way home Lindsay told me her wrist hurt. We weren't too concerned, since she was due for a month's rest from pitching anyway.

Top pitchers typically throw for eleven months of the year, taking only August off. For years people thought the natural underhand windmill softball motion didn't hurt the arm, unlike the less natural overhand throwing motion of baseball pitchers. This is partly true. It isn't unusual for top pitchers to throw three or four games in a weekend tournament. Even college coaches will routinely allow their ace to pitch both games of key doubleheaders. We found out too late, though, that overuse can definitely cause problems. In early September it was time for Lindsay to begin working out for her last high school season. But when she tried to pitch, or even throw the ball overhand, her wrist really hurt.

After a couple of trips to the doctor and to an orthopedic specialist, and eight more weeks of rest, she was diagnosed with a deep bone bruise on the tip of her radius. She started a long rehabilitation project with a physical therapist. Even when the pain finally disappeared, Lindsay's pitching and overhand throwing mechanics were not right. During her entire senior season she was only able to play as a desig-nated hitter. She was still a top hitter, but not being able to pitch or play first base ate at her, and at me as well. Of all the stressors, this bothered me the most. Any parent hates to see their child suffer. And there wasn't a thing I could do to make it better. ***Strike three. Third out. No runs, no hits, no errors. Lots of stress.***

So, in the year before I spotted the lump in my leg I had so much stress added to my life that I would wake up at night and wouldn't even know what to worry about first. It was the only time in my life that I ever suffered from insomnia. There's no doubt in my mind that my usually robust immune system was weakened to the point that it couldn't protect me. Cancer gained a foothold.

10

Chemo

10/18/01

Dear Family, Friends, Shipmates, Classmates, Argonauts, and IHMCers,

Its chemotherapy time again. Today was the second of the three days of this round of the big guns. (I look at the ankle surgery as establishing air supremacy. Now we call in the precision weapons.) After tomorrow, I'll have two rounds down and four more to go. I decided to send a SITREP this afternoon instead of waiting until completion of the treatment. Based on last month's experience, I'll be too wiped out by tomorrow to write anything remotely creative, entertaining, or maybe even coherent.

Actually, this round has been relatively easy so far. My reading and my cancer warrior friends tell me that the second (and third if you're lucky) rounds are almost "vacation" rounds. You know what to expect, and you haven't built up a chemical level that weakens your own cells too much. As of today I've just experienced minor side effects—a little queasy from time to time, and a general pooped feeling that's complicated, or maybe caused, by mild insomnia. The nurses told me this morning that the antiemetic that combats nausea can cause wakefulness. If that's the case, it's an easy choice to make. I'd rather be awake in bed than awake hugging the porcelain throne!

Before the session yesterday I was weighed and measured. While the typical chemo patient has trouble keeping their weight up, I actually GAINED four pounds in the last month. I guess that shouldn't have surprised me. Nurse Nancy is an excellent cook who gives me plenty of healthy variety. Plus, my appetite is good. Even though the chemicals definitely affect how food tastes, I still eat plenty. I attribute that to Navy training. My former shipmates will tell you that regardless of what kind of mystery meat was being served in the Dirty Shirt wardroom, and despite the fact the vegetables were "cooked with nuclear power" until they all had approximately the same flavor and baby-food consistency, I always cleaned my tray before hitting the autodog machine. Plus, the ankle prohibits much in the way of aerobic exercise. My body was used to 5-6 days per week in the gym or on a bike, so my calorie burn rate is way down.

My only problem at the moment is the damn Yankees. Here I am, working hard to manage stress, and Joe Torre's boys fight their way back against the A's by winning 3 straight. That's as stressful for a Yankee-hater like me as it is for the Yankee-lovers like Swayk and my dad. As much as I hate the Yanks, I've got to admire them. Jeter and Mussina and even Clemens are amazing ballplayers—supported by a team that does whatever it takes.

For the Volts—Roo goes along to chemo sessions to keep me company. There's no fence to hang him on, so he sits in my chair. Maybe I should hang him up on an IV stand so he can have his normal bird's-eye view.

GO USA! Larry

I was in charge of the Navy's METOC budget during the heat of the Clinton administration's defense downsizing. As America tried to claim a premature peace dividend, we were faced with continual budget cuts and threats of cuts. I tried to remind everyone to keep a positive attitude as we fought to do our jobs without nearly enough money or people. On the white board in my office, I wrote in big red letters,

The pain is MANDATORY, but the suffering is OPTIONAL.

You can put a positive spin on defense budget cuts, but in chemotherapy both the pain <u>and</u> the suffering are mandatory. Every chemo patient suffers.

SITREP #13

10/24/01

Dear Family, Friends, Shipmates, Classmates, Argonauts, and IHMCers,

Today is a notable day in my "war." For the first time since September 8th the lovely Nurse Nancy has left me on my own. I can drive and walk easily now, and the worst side effects of chemo cycle #2 have worn off. After yes-

terday's ankle check-up with Dr. Mike, I sent her back to Mandeville for a few days while I remained in Pensacola. She has to get the mail, make sure the house is ready for showing, do a lot of laundry, and make sure the bills are paid. That's a full time job, even when you aren't providing custom in-home nursing care.

Coincidentally, last night was the first night in a month that didn't have a football game or a baseball playoff game to watch. So after dinner I popped in a videotape of BULL DURHAM (hey, you can't just quit cold turkey!) and went to bed early.

I spoke too soon in the last SITREP when I said round 2 of chemo might be a relative vacation. And I shouldn't have likened chemo to precision weapons, either. There's WAY too much collateral damage! Actually, it lies somewhere between William Tecumseh Sherman's scorched earth March to the Sea and low-yield tactical nuclear weapons (thanks, Ed, for the proper analogy). I don't think I can adequately describe the 24-hour period at the end. Imagine the planet's worst tequila hangover combined with other-side-of-the-world jet lag. But, we're now "two down and four to go."

I have blood work on Friday morning. Then Lindsay and I will drive to LA for the weekend. It's homecoming at FHS and it will be her first trip back since she came to college in August.

A real autumn cold front will move through Pensacola tomorrow, so I figured I would take advantage of today's humid low-80s and go sit on the beach. I worked until my stamina gave out this afternoon, rested a bit, then drove out to Pensacola Beach with a chair, a book, and a couple of Abita Ambers in a cooler. On some days, this convalescent leave isn't too shabby!

GO USA! Larry

Describing chemotherapy to someone who has never experienced it is a bit like a new mother trying to describe labor and delivery to a man. We men know that labor must be very tough, but we will never really, fully understand. Cheryl Shank says it is like the difference between going to a bullfight and being the matador in the ring.

When it comes to describing chemo, Lance Armstrong's chemotherapy chapter is the best one I read. The future Tour de France champion (he won his fourth in a row in 2002) needed all his determination and stamina to survive four debilitating chemo cycles in 1996. I read

Armstrong's chemo chapter multiple times. Shortly after cycle three, I found myself nodding my head in agreement and shaking my head in sympathy as I read it again. I thought Lance had the chemotherapy experience nailed. But then it hit me. The first time I read that particular chapter, it was just two days before my first trip to Chemoland. Naturally, I took my time and read it closely and concentrated on every detail, because I really wanted to get an idea of what I was in for. But even though I certainly paid attention the first time through, it wasn't until I had survived a few cycles that I could fully appreciate what Lance had suffered.

◆   ◆   ◆

From September 2001 through early February 2002, the Chemo Calendar governed my life. For chemo patients, the calendar isn't divided into months or weeks, but into chemotherapy cycles. In my treatment regimen, each cycle began with Day One, and lasted from three to four weeks. Then I started over at Day One. Most of the time it didn't matter to me what day of the week it was, or even what month. I didn't care about holidays, only where they fell on the chemo calendar. At one point I remember having to think hard for a few minutes before I could figure out what month it really was!

Each chemo cycle began with a visit to Dr. Tan's office. After weighing me and taking my vital signs, a nurse would draw a blood sample for a complete blood count. Dr. Tan reviewed the counts of red and white blood cells, hemoglobin and hematocrit (used to measure oxygen-carrying capacity), platelets (clotting ability), and neutrophils (the portion of the white blood cells critical for fighting infection). He gave me a quick exam and asked me to describe my reactions and side effects of the previous cycle. Then he discussed our plan and scheduled the next cycle.

From the exam room, Nancy and I headed down the hall to the treatment room. That's where a small family of cancer warriors gathers to suffer together every day. A dozen recliners and other big chairs line the walls, each with their own IV stand. A diverse group of patients come and go. I found amazing strength and willpower in that group. Even the oldest, sickest, and weakest patients would invariably summon a depth of courage to smile and encourage others. When a patient finally finishes their last chemo treatment, the standard farewell in the treatment room is, "Goodbye. Good luck. And I hope I never see you again…in here."

On Day One I received three bags of intravenous fluid. The first was an anti-nausea drug. The second was carboplatin, a platinum-based chemotherapy drug, and the third drug in the cocktail was VP-16, a version of the chemotherapy drug etoposide. Doses are calculated based on an estimate of the patient's body surface area. At 6'4" I cover a lot of surface, so my doses were pretty large. On Day Two I got the nausea prophylactic and etoposide. Twenty-four hours later I dragged myself back into Sacred Heart for one more dose of etoposide. Each cycle, I began to feel tired on Day Two, and by the end of the treatment on Day Three, I was flat-out exhausted. It took days to begin to recover.

At the Naval Academy, the period from the end of Christmas leave until the beginning of spring is known in Bancroft Hall as The Dark Ages. The name accurately describes the amount of daylight, the winter weather in Annapolis, and the mood of the Brigade. For me, Days 3 through 7 on the chemo calendar were The Dark Days. In every one of my cycles, Day 4 was the darkest. Beginning around Day 7 or 8, most of the side effects began to diminish to manageable levels. The farther away I got from Day 4, the better my life as a chemo patient became.

◆　　　◆　　　◆

Before I started my first chemotherapy session, a very pleasant nurse sat down with me to go over a long list of possible side effects. The sheet they use at Hematology and Oncology Associates has thirty-nine potential side effects, listed in three columns. It's too bad it isn't like a Chinese restaurant, where you pick one from column A, one from column B, and one from column C. Instead, it's a buffet. You are required to sample from a whole lot of dishes. My drug combination of carboplatin and etoposide rated checkmarks in twenty-three of the blocks. Fortunately, I didn't experience all 23, but I did bat way over .500.

Chemotherapy works by attacking and destroying fast-growing cells. Cells growing and reproducing out of control characterize cancer. While many cancers respond to chemo, some types, such as prostate cancer, have cells that don't grow quite as fast. Therefore, they aren't treatable with chemo. Chemo causes so many undesirable side effects because many normal body cells also grow rapidly. The drugs that are attacking the cancer also destroy stomach, mouth, and intestinal linings, hair, and bone marrow cells. They can weaken muscles and affect lung and kidney tissues.

Fortunately, oncologists have greatly refined the chemo cocktails over the years. The drugs I took were much more selective than those available a generation ago. Consequently, the severity of side effects is somewhat less than it used to be. I sure am glad of that, because what I experienced was plenty unpleasant!

Chemotherapy may have saved my life, but I still hate it. I certainly hope I live to see the day that chemotherapy is nothing more than a curiosity of medical history. In a hundred years, I predict it will be thought of as a truly barbaric approach. However, it is one of the few reliable treatment options currently available. And it does work.

◆   ◆   ◆

Oncologists and cancer nurses are big fans of blood samples. It seems that every time they see you they want to relieve you of some of your blood. The chemo patient's Complete Blood Count governs the dose and timing of each chemo cycle. Plus, it lets the professionals know if you are in danger of becoming anemic or of having your immune system completely debilitated.

During each cycle I would have a CBC on Day One and again around Day 11. After each of the first two cycles, Dr. Tan ordered two interim CBCs—one on Day 10 to see how low my counts fell, and another on Day 13 to make sure the bone marrow was beginning to recover enough to bring my counts back up toward normal. Once he was confident that I would not have major blood count problems, we went to just two blood draws per cycle.

The nurses' interest in each CBC raised my scientific curiosity. I asked them to give me printouts each time. I made graphs of the key numbers. Red blood cells, hemoglobin, and hematocrit measure your blood's ability to move oxygen from the lungs throughout the body. If your counts fall too low in these categories, you suffer from anemia. Then (if you happen to have a cute three-year old grandson) you can try out for a role in a Procrit commercial. Platelets are the part of the blood that causes it to clot. If your platelet count falls too low you can suffer excessive bruising or bleeding.

The most common, and potentially most serious, blood-related side effect is the weakening of the immune system. White blood cells are the infection fighters, especially the ones called neutrophils. Usually, about half your white blood cells are neutrophils. Oncologists expect the number of these cells to decrease as a result of chemotherapy. But if they get too low, they must delay chemotherapy until the patient's immune system regains at least a minimal robustness.

While at first glance it may seem like a good idea to delay treatment and have a longer period of rest and recovery before the chemo train hits you again, the object of chemotherapy is to keep re-attacking the cancer cells before they have time to recover and start growing again. The doctor times the cycles to try to achieve a balance that maximizes damage to cancer cells and minimizes damage to healthy cells.

The range for a normal neutrophil count is 2,200 to 4,800 (neutrophils per microliter of blood). If your count remains below a thousand, you probably won't be able to begin your next cycle on time. At the beginning of my first cycle of chemo, my count was at the upper end of the normal range. During each cycle it would fall well below normal, then climb slowly back upward. By Day One of the next cycle, it would "peak" at a level high enough to allow further treatment. By the end of cycle three, I could only recover to a peak count of 2,200—the bottom limit of the normal range. From then until the end of chemo, my bacteria-fighting cells were weak and far below the infection-preventing threshold number.

Similarly, the total white blood cell count bottomed out lower each cycle, and recovered to lower and lower levels in between. Even by March, a full seven weeks after the last day of chemo, my blood counts had only barely gotten back into the basement level of the normal range. Fortunately, I never suffered any serious infections during my chemo time. I did have an ingrown toenail that became infected while I was in the hospital in September. Despite regular soaking and treatment, it took until April to clear it up. The only other noticeable impact of my weakened immune system were a handful of pimple-like infected hair follicles that would appear on my thighs and hips between Days 12 and 16 of every cycle.

◆   ◆   ◆

Hair loss is the most visible side effect of chemotherapy. It is less of an issue for most men than for women. With shaved heads and very short haircuts in style, I wasn't really worried about losing my hair. I was almost anxious to see what I looked like without it. Hair started falling out a couple of weeks into cycle one. For two weeks it fell like autumn leaves in a strong wind. Every time I scratched or rubbed my head I would have a handful of hairs. But when it got thinned out to a scant peach fuzz-like covering, it suddenly stopped falling out. A friend figured that since chemo only attacks fast-growing cells, my remaining hairs must be slow growing. Nancy set the hair clippers on their shortest setting and buzzed the peach fuzz to about an eighth of an inch. I was hoping for a grizzled old Marine look, but I came up with something closer to Curly Howard of the Three Stooges.

The hair on the rest of my body also thinned or disappeared. Some places it was gone completely, others it just thinned out a little. The places that were shaved for the surgeries in September remained pretty much hairless until chemo was over. You don't realize the value of hair until it's gone. In addition to keeping your head warm, it is meant to serve as a good dry lubricant. When it's not there, body parts stick and chafe. For example, if you rub your nose, your nostrils stick. Now this might be a pretty funny trick if you're out drinking beer with the guys, but it's rather inconvenient in a meeting or at the dinner table.

I looked at hair loss as just another part of the cancer experience. But nausea and vomiting were the side effects I feared most. That horrible sick stomach feeling is something with which most everyone can identify. I had read and heard awful stories of what other cancer warriors have suffered. Fortunately, modern antiemetic drugs prevented vomiting and greatly limited nausea for me. I did have a persistent queasiness that never quite went away, but I learned to live with that. Navy buddy Sean Memmen made a hydrographic survey trip to Italy during my chemo. He brought back a bottle of "digestivo," a rather terrible tasting Italian bitters that I always found excellent for an upset stomach. It helped calm the queasiness.

Actually, I not only maintained my weight throughout the chemo regimen, I gained between five and ten pounds over the five months of treatment. My appetite was good except for the first of the Dark Days. Certainly, the weight gain was partly due to limited exercise. Before cancer I worked out five or six days a week. Surgery put an abrupt end to my exercise. By the time my ankle was strong enough to resume useful activity, chemo had pretty much sapped my strength and energy.

My sense of taste was definitely affected. During the Dark Days, everything tasted like it had been dusted with powdered aluminum. Even though I didn't feel like eating anything for several days, I found that having food in my stomach lessened the cramps and queasiness. Nancy cooked potato soup, scrambled eggs and baked potatoes to keep me going. I found that using plastic utensils helped lessen the metallic taste.

Coffee was the hardest adjustment of all. I am an unrepentant caffeine addict. In my sea duty days, shipboard coffee was considered naval personnel fuel. There was always a pot on the warmer in the wardroom. By 4:00 am, at the end of the midwatch, it was so burned and strong that you worried about putting a spoon in the mug. We drank it anyway. The Chief Petty Officers, with their years of experience, would order extra coffee before the ship was scheduled for a shipyard overhaul. They would lock up cans of ground coffee in their division storerooms. You could get a lot of extra work done in the shipyard if you had a five-pound can of coffee to trade.

These days, I normally start my morning with my own version of a home-brewed latte. I use a fancy little machine to make a pot of strong European espresso and add hot skim milk. By the time I get to work, I'm at full speed! When I went through the full day of my first surgery on September 10 without coffee, it was undoubtedly the first time in my adult life. As my surgery was delayed until later and later in the day, the caffeine headache didn't help my impatience to get going. I tried to bribe the pre-op nurses into giving me a cup of java. They refused. I think they just wanted me to go to sleep so they could save on the anesthetics.

While in the hospital, I drank Navy coffee with breakfast, and then asked Nancy to buy me a latte from the hospital's Java Joe shop later in the morning. After a few days she decided to make it herself rather than pay the outrageous coffee shop price. After the first chemo cycle, I sensed a problem. My favorite caffeine source did not taste right! First I accused Nancy of making it wrong. Eventually it dawned on me that my chemo-altered stomach and taste buds didn't like coffee anymore. During the Dark Days, I couldn't drink it at all.

But the caffeine withdrawal headaches, on top of the chemo side effects, were too much. Again my Navy friends came to the rescue. Two officers who worked with me when I was the Director of the National Ice Center were working together in the METOC Facility in Naples, Italy. Lisa Frailey was the Commanding Officer and Tim Rush was her Executive Officer. They sent me a couple of boxes of my favorite Italian candy. Curiously, its name is in English—Pocket Coffee. They are espresso-filled chocolates. A couple of those in the morning provided my caffeine fix during the Dark Days.

Coffee wasn't the only thing that didn't taste the same during chemo. My desire for carbonated drinks like beer and Diet Coke disappeared. Late in the cycles I would occasionally drink one or the other, but I didn't enjoy them nearly as much as usual. Fortunately, water and orange juice still tasted pretty good. That's important, because it's absolutely critical for chemo patients to stay well hydrated. Drinking plenty of water helps protect the kidneys from chemo damage. It's also possible that it mollifies the stomach-related side effects. Some studies have found that Vitamin C also reduces chemo stomach problems. Plus, it is a powerful cancer fighter on its own. So I drank glass after glass of water and OJ during the Dark Days and continued pumping fluids throughout the chemo regimen.

Thankfully, I was able to avoid the lip and mouth sores that plague some chemo warriors. Instead, my body's reaction was to start each cycle with spasms of hiccups. Hiccups were not one of the 39 potential side effects on the "you may experience some discomfort" list. How about that? I even got a bonus side effect! After the hiccups stopped, I produced buckets of thick mucous in my throat. During the Dark Days, I spent a substantial part of my waking hours hiccupping, coughing, and hacking.

I have never had a very sensitive sense of smell. Maybe it's because I spent too many years inhaling fumes from marine diesel and jet fuels. Chemo changed that—and not in a good way. Early in the cycle, any odor at all would turn my stomach. If I ever have to take chemotherapy again, I'm going to campaign for a Constitutional Amendment to ban perfumes and aftershaves. Even normally good smells—like towels right out of the drier, fresh-brewed coffee, or a new bar of Irish Spring—were overpoweringly unpleasant.

Chemo affected all five of my senses. Changes in taste and smell were the most unpleasant, but touch, sight and hearing all reacted as well. It brought back long-buried memories of hangovers I suffered once or twice in my young and stupid days. During the Dark Days, I didn't want to look at bright lights or hear any loud or sharp sounds. If Nancy banged a pan on the stove or put her coffee cup down too hard on the glass table she earned a pathetic moan from me. A line from one of my very first Jimmy Buffett favorites kept running through my head. "My head hurts, my feet stink, and I don't love Jesus (but if I don't die by Thursday, I'll be roaring Friday night)."

I spent the Dark Days communicating with grunts and moans. I was too tired to take the trouble to form my clouded thoughts into words or phrases, much less complete sentences. The fatigue that weighed so heavily after each cycle was the most discouraging part of the whole experience. I refused to talk on the phone. I didn't want to depress or worry people, but I couldn't muster the energy to be upbeat or polite. I didn't want any company, except Nancy. She put up with my whining and complaining and was a tower of strength. I'm sure she was tempted to tell me to shut up and suck it up, but she was too kind. I'm sure I would have just moaned and ignored her anyway.

On the potential side effects score sheet, both constipation and diarrhea had check marks next to them. Now, at first glance, I wasn't concerned. I guess everyone has experience with these two from time to time. Surely I would not have to endure *both* of them? I thought that would be cruel and unusual punishment. Why not a nice simple combination that would mean no problems? But the sheet was right. You, lucky cancer patient, can have both! Early on, the drugs shut everything down. I found pitted prunes to be an acquired taste—especially if they are flavored with powdered aluminum. Later in the cycle, after your stomach and intestinal lining cells have been destroyed, you shift to the other extreme. Uggh.

Even though the physical side effects were bad enough, the worst part of chemotherapy for me is what it did to my mind. During the Dark Days, I just didn't give a _____ about anything. (Fill in the blank with the word or phrase that is most descriptive for you.) I just plain did not care! I guess this was a chemical-induced depression, but for me it was a horrible feeling. I've never lacked enthusiasm in my life. The first cycle or two, I was afraid that my mind would be permanently altered. Every time, it was a relief to wake up on Day 7 or 8 and care about life again!

When the Dark Days ended and the depression went away, the most unpleasant side effects diminished. Then the last one would start. Each cycle I would develop a couple of small patches of dry, flaking skin. Despite regular, frequent lotion drenching, the end result was always a painful, burning itch that persisted for a couple of days.

In retrospect, it seems like I spent my five months in chemo as one long, frequently interrupted trip to the bathroom. If I wasn't trying to ease stomach cramps, I was getting a drink or recycling fluids, or I was coughing up a lung, or I was scratching some place you can't scratch in public.

◆　　　◆　　　◆

Actually, I tolerated chemo much better than most of my fellow patients. Throughout the treatment regimen, people were surprised at how healthy I looked. And for a flabby, weak, and tired guy, I felt great—once the Dark Days were over. Still, in my memory, each one of those six chemotherapy cycles would individually qualify as the toughest thing I ever went through in my life. Putting them together just means the toughest six things I ever had to do all happened in one twenty-week period.

Before cancer, I would sometimes get out of the shower and admire myself in the bathroom mirror. I wasn't going to win any magazine cover contracts, but at 6'4" and 205 pounds, I was in pretty good shape. I even had a hint of abdominal muscles. I would flex and congratulate myself on being "not bad for 48 years old." One day during cycle three, I looked at myself in the mirror and started laughing out loud.

Looking back was this strange looking fellow with random hairless patches; a puzzle piece missing from his lower right leg; a color test swatch from Barbie's home decorating kit on his left thigh; a matching pair of purple zippers on the right groin; a soft, bloated belly; and what looked like half a golf ball imbedded under the skin below his left collarbone. He was topped off with a fuzzy head that looked like a failed Chia pet—or an albino kiwi. And he was laughing at me.

11

Paradise on Earth

SITREP #14

10/31/01

Dear Family, Friends, Shipmates, Classmates, Argonauts, and IHMCers,

Happy Halloween, everyone.

I'm happy to report that I'm a contributing officer in the Navy once again. Since I'm on medical hold and can't retire until treatment is complete, and since the second half of each chemo cycle has ten to fifteen good days, it was time to find a way to earn my keep. The Chief of Naval Education and Training (CNET) is headquartered in Pensacola. Since both the METOC folks at Stennis and the University of West Florida work closely with CNET, it was a logical place to offer my skills. I am working with Task Force EXCEL helping to bring about the Navy's Revolution in Training. When I met CAPT Vince Lynch, CNET's TF EXCEL director, we recognized each other. We were both Seventh Company Seadogs at USNA in 1971-72. He was a firstie when I was a plebe. Once again, it's a small Navy—even 30 years later.

But before I really get back to work, Nancy and I are taking some leave for a long-planned trip to Hawaii for Ty Aldinger's retirement. Charlie and Ty are the kind of people that make our Navy and our country great. We planned our own "retirement vacation trip" so we could attend Ty's celebration. Fortunately, the chemo cycle cooperated. Stamina and resistance to infections are down, but otherwise I'm doing well. But even more fortunately, Nancy doesn't mind traveling with someone who poops out at 9:00 every evening and can't stand shopping. But hey, I was like that even before chemotherapy!

Aloha and GO USA! Larry

Nancy and I have made a multitude of absolutely wonderful friends during our married life and our Navy career. Our lives would be much poorer without any of them, but if we were forced to make a short list, Ty and Charlie Aldinger would probably eke out the top spot. I am proud to make the statement that Ty Aldinger is my best friend. But I'm sure that I'm not the only person who claims Ty as his best friend. He has all those qualities that make him a best-friend type of guy. He and Charlie (only telemarketers call her Charleen) have shared a number of duty stations with us, going back to our Masters Degree work at the Naval Postgraduate School in Monterey, CA in 1978–79.

Ty was one year ahead of me at the Naval Academy and we became METOC specialists at the same time. He was one of our top candidates for the admiral selection in 2000. Had I been in charge of the selection board, he would have been my choice. But I sure am glad he wasn't picked. Now, that may sound like a funny thing to say about your best friend, but consider my reasoning. Had he become my new boss, I would have gladly remained in the Chief of Staff job. Considering the unbelievable schedule in the METOC headquarters, and without impending retirement to goad me into seeing the doctor, my cancer would have had many more months to run rampant through my body before I did something about it.

As it turned out, neither of us was chosen, and we both decided to wrap up our active duty careers in 2001 and move on to the exciting civilian world. At my retirement ceremony in May, Nancy told Ty that we were going to be in Hawaii for his November festivities "no matter what." She challenged fate a little bit there, but it worked out fine.

◆   ◆   ◆

When we met with Dr. Tan at the beginning of chemo cycle #2, he proposed starting cycle #3 during the first week in November. We told him about our trip plans, and he agreed that we could travel as scheduled. So we pushed cycle #3 back a few days. I certainly was not traveling under ideal physical conditions. My immune system was much weaker than normal. I figured there was a very high probability that I would come down with a cold after fighting the airport terminal and security line crowds and breathing the recycled airplane air for so many hours. I had very limited stamina. Most people don't fly to Hawaii to take afternoon naps, but they were important highlights of my vacation. My ankle was reasonably strong by November, but it still hurt after a modest time either standing or walking. I was still fighting significant swelling of the right foot and lower leg. But at least I was off the crutches. And above all, we weren't in Hawaii to take care of the physical self. We were there to celebrate with friends. It was a trip for the mental and spiritual sides. The body was just going to have to suck it up and keep up for as long as possible.

Charlie was our island tour guide for the week. She shifted the tour schedule whenever I ran out of gas. Actually, I didn't wind down and slowly come to a stop. It was more like running into a wall. I would feel great and be full of energy, then suddenly everything would start to hurt all at once, and I would begin to whine. Nap time! It must have been like traveling with a baby.

◆   ◆   ◆

Like Nancy, Charlie Aldinger could teach a graduate course in being a great Navy spouse. Back in the 1980s, when Navy husbands were still a rarity, we had a slogan: **Navy Wife—the toughest job in the Navy!** It still applies. Navy wives have an amazingly flexible ability to pick up the household and family, pack everything away and arrange for shots, passports, and tickets to set up a new home anywhere in the world. When the family arrives at the new duty station, the Sailor is immediately thrown into the hustle of the new job—often departing soon after for days, weeks, or months at sea. The active duty member has immediate access to medical, dental, banking, and postal services. Plus, he has a built-in social group of new and old friends. If his new ship is deploying overseas, he has a comforting (if tiring) routine at sea and exciting foreign ports to help take his mind off the separation from his family. He gets the welcome chance to do the job for which he has been training for so many months.

The spouse, on the other hand, has to unpack everything and set up the new home. She has to register the kids for school and find a church, day care, a doctor, a dentist, scout troops, a bank, and stores in a town where she doesn't know her way around. She has to get the car, washing machine, or lawn mower repaired when they break down. Invariably, the appliances time their demise for the week after the ship gets under way. She may have Navy friends in town, but the children probably don't yet know anyone. Is there any question why the spouse's job is tougher? Either Nancy or Charlie could teach the course…and use the other as a role model.

◆   ◆   ◆

Ty and Charlie had two tours of duty in Hawaii, one before their daughters were born, and then a return to Paradise for Ty's last two Navy jobs—as commanding officer of the Pacific METOC organization, and finally as the METOC officer on the Pacific Fleet staff. They were the last two stops in a long and notable career. As the head of all Navy METOC activities in the huge Pacific theater, he had to close our center on Guam as part of the response to a congressionally mandated base realignment and closure law. Ty developed a plan that saved taxpayer dollars and actually increased our service to the fleet in the Pacific. As a reward, the Navy kept him in command an extra year so he could complete the reorganization. I suspect that we really wanted to have someone to blame if his aggressive plan failed. Actually, we knew that if anyone could make it happen smoothly, it was Ty.

Among the many plaques and presentations at retirement, a Naval officer traditionally receives a "shadow box" from his last wardroom. Our nautical superstition holds that it is bad luck for a sailor's shadow to leave the ship before him. To prevent misfortune, we give our retiring shipmate a container to capture his shadow, so it can safely be carried ashore for the last time. It is a usually a beautiful wood and glass box containing an American flag, the officer's medals and decorations, and an engraved brass plate listing all of his duty assignments. Ty added a thoughtful and wonderful touch to his retirement ceremony by presenting Charlie with a matching shadow box. Her job history was longer than his! Among her many other talents, Charlie is a terrific writer. When they lived in Louisiana, she worked in public relations for the New Orleans Museum of Art. It was fun to hear Charlie's clever advertising copy on the radio as Ty and I carpooled to Mississippi. She now has a great position as the public relations director for the Honolulu Academy of Arts.

With Charlie finally able to settle into one job for more than a year or two, and with daughters Stacy and Kelly thriving at the Punahou School, the Aldingers never even considered leaving Hawaii. They found a gorgeous lot in the heart of the Manoa Valley and built their dream home. The lanai, which Ty nicknamed the Tree House, is surrounded by lush tropical vegetation, and overlooks the narrow, rushing Manoa River. The first time we sat down out there, with the trade winds blowing down the valley, birds singing, and intermittent five-minute long "Manoa-sunshine" rain showers falling through the trees, I told Charlie that I may never leave. She still may wake up some morning to find me camped in the corner of the Tree House. She'll just have to clean around me.

Ty's retirement ceremony was held aboard the battleship MISSOURI. In 1945 the grand old lady was the setting for the surrender ceremony in Tokyo Bay that ended World War II. She is now on display on battleship row in Pearl Harbor, right next to the USS ARIZONA Memorial. The setting and the people made it the most memorable retirement ceremony of the many I've attended in my career. Ty gave me the honor of reading the poem "Old Glory" as a folded American flag was slowly and reverently passed from member to member of an Honor Color Guard, and finally to him. It is an emotional piece for me, and reading it just a few weeks after 9/11 made it a real challenge. My voice was shaking by the time I reached the last paragraph.

Old Glory

I am the flag of the United States of America.
My name is Old Glory.
I fly atop the world's tallest buildings.
I stand watch in America's halls of justice.
I fly majestically over great institutions of learning.
I stand guard with the greatest military power in
the world.
Look up and see me!

I stand for peace—honor—truth—and justice.
I stand for freedom.
I am confident.
I am arrogant.
I am proud.

When I am flown with my fellow banners,
My head is a little higher,
My colors a little truer.
I bow to no one.

I am recognized all over the world.
I am worshipped.
I am loved.
And I am feared.

I have fought in every battle of every major war for
more than 200 years:
Gettysburg, Shiloh, Appomattox, San Juan Hill, The
Trenches of France,

The Argonne Forest, Anzio, Rome, The Beaches of
Normandy, Guam,
Okinawa, Japan, Korea, Viet Nam, in the Persian
Gulf, Afghanistan,
And a score of places long forgotten by all but
those who were there with me.
I was there!

I led my Sailors, Airmen, Marines, and Soldiers.
I followed them and watched over them.
They loved me.

I was on a small hill on Iwo Jima.
I was dirty, battle worn, and tired.
But my Marines and Soldiers cheered me!
And I was proud!

I have been soiled, burned, torn, and trampled on
the streets of countries
That I have helped set free.
It does not hurt—for I am invincible.

I have been soiled, burned, torn, and trampled on
the streets of my own country.
When it is by those whom I have served with in
battle—
It hurts.

But I have overcome.
For I am strong!
I have slipped the bonds of earth,
And from my vantage point on the moon,
I stand watch over the uncharted new frontiers of
space.

I have been silent witness to all of America's finest
hours.
But my finest hour comes when I am torn in strips
to be used as bandages
For my wounded companions on the field of battle.
Or when I fly at half-mast to honor
My Sailors, My Soldiers, My Airmen, My Marines,
and
When I lie in the trembling arms of a grieving
mother,
At the graveside of her fallen son or daughter.

I am proud!
My name is Old Glory.
Long may I wave, Dear God!
Long may I wave!

We had a fabulous week in Hawaii. Every night was party night at
Ty and Charlie's house, since Nancy and I were just two of the small
multitude of houseguests they entertained that week. One was Ty's 83-
year old Aunt Edith from Florida. This beautiful bundle of energy calls
herself "the last leaf on the tree" from her generation of the family. She
is an absolutely delightful person. Another guest was "Auntie" Muriel,
who flew out from California. She and her husband were Ty's neighbors in Carmel when he and Charlie began dating in 1977. She's
become a great friend to a whole generation of METOC officers. Cancer took Muriel's husband Dan just a few years ago, so she was very
understanding of the task ahead of Nancy and the mental and emotional demands she would have to meet.

   The youngest houseguest was Ensign Kenny Vargas, one of Charlie's distant cousins, who took a few days leave for the trip to the
islands. Kenny had been an enlisted Navy dental technician when Ty
inspired him to seek a career as a Naval Officer. With the help of the
GI bill, he earned a college degree and engineering certification. Then
he turned down attractive civilian offers to return to uniform via

Officer Candidate School. It sure is reassuring to know that I left "my Navy" in good hands.

◆   ◆   ◆

The Warrenfeltz family has known Stacy and Kelly Aldinger for all of their young lives. When Charlie was newly pregnant with Kelly, she spent a few weeks with us in Monterey, along with Stacy, who had just turned two. Charlie was beginning yet another new job while Ty was finishing his tour on the aircraft carrier USS ENTERPRISE before his transfer to join me at our weather supercomputer center. Poor Charlie was fighting morning sickness and Stacy missed her father. Ty had been away at sea for too much of her young life. Since my khaki uniform reminded her of Daddy, we became good buddies.

I had a nice garden behind our house. Stacy helped me water the tomatoes, peppers and beans every day. It was a long walk down the hill for a two-year old. Unfortunately, after we turned on the hose, it was far too long a walk back up the hill for a two-year old who was just starting potty training! My string beans were ready for harvest while Charlie and Stacy were our guests. The problem was I had greatly underestimated how many beans my plants would produce. Charlie swears I even served string beans for breakfast one morning. To this day, Stacy won't eat them.

The following February, on the Sunday morning Kelly was born, I got the call to baby-sit Stacy. The poor kid had the flu. She awoke feeling absolutely horrible and found Uncle Larry in her house instead of the Mommy she really, really wanted. We still laugh about how she threw up all over me and gave me the flu the day her sister was born. Maybe it was the flu. Maybe it was a payback for all the string beans.

Stacy and Kelly have grown into absolutely wonderful kids. They are mature, smart, athletic, loving, funny, talented, and kind. They are leaders in their church, their water polo and cross-country teams, and in their school. They comfortably played host to the many guests who showed up for the retirement week festivities. They twisted my arm just a little to get me to sing one of their childhood favorites—*There was an Old Lady Who Swallowed a Fly*—for video camera posterity. Then they topped my performance with their two-woman rendition of the "So Long, Farewell, auf Wiedersehen, Goodnight" scene from *The Sound of Music*. The Aldinger family has an enviable quality that is all too rare—parents who are proud of their kids, and kids who are proud of their parents.

SITREP #15

11/10/01

Dear Family, Friends, Shipmates, Classmates, Argonauts, and IHMCers,

Nancy and I are trying to do our part to support the tourist economy. We spent the past week in Hawaii. As I write this early on Saturday morning, we're sitting in the San Francisco airport USO. The oncoming National Guard watch section stopped in for breakfast a few minutes ago. I don't know if camouflaged soldiers with M-16s will deter terrorists. I don't know if they will make the public more comfortable when we fly. But I guess it is one small security measure the country can take. Air travel is certainly harder than it was a few months ago. Flight consolidations left us with long layovers on the west coast in both directions. Lines throughout the airport are certainly longer. Our former carefree approach to life is curtailed as we attempt to balance our love of liberty and our need for risk-reducing restrictions.

The weekend version of the Today Show covered ENTERPRISE's return to Norfolk this morning. It's a small Navy. We saw the wife and children of Big E's Oceanographer making welcome home signs. Cindy was our command ombudsman when Ken was with me at NAVOCEANO. She is a leader among the Enterprise battlegroup families, too.

Our trip was a memorable R&R interlude in the cancer war. A week with wonderful friends in Paradise on Earth is great medicine for whatever ails you. It recharged my spirit and mind. In addition to the many friends at Ty Aldinger's memorable retirement on board the battleship MISSOURI, there were a lot of people from the Naval Oceanographic Office in Honolulu for the OCEANS 2001 convention. The NAVO family is a wonderful, supportive group. Now it is time to make our way back to Pensacola to begin Chemo Cycle #3 on Monday.

GO USA! Larry

Ty helped organize the Marine Technology Society's OCEANS 2001 conference. The U.S. OCEANS series, co-hosted by the Institute of Electrical and Electronics Engineers, is held in a different city each year. It is one of the primary oceanography meetings, especially for people who work in the at-sea end of the business. With an eight-ship fleet of military survey vessels operating all over the world, the Naval Oceanographic Office is a big fish in the at-sea oceanography business and usually has a fairly large presence at the OCEANS conference. It was one of the things I tried to encourage strongly when I was the commanding officer of NAVO. Sending a large contingent to a conference is expensive, but I think it is a good investment. It encouraged our scientists to advance their personal academic interests, allowed them to make important contacts in the science, and reminded the oceanography world that NAVO has been a leader in marine science and technology for 170 years.

One of the highlights of OCEANS 2001 was a reception hosted by Admiral Thomas Fargo (then the Commander in Chief of the Pacific Fleet) on board a NAVO survey ship, the USNS SUMNER. Security concerns kept the ship in a distant corner of the Navy base for most of the week, but she was allowed to move pierside near the Aloha Tower in downtown Honolulu for the reception. Nancy and I were thrilled to see the professionalism, pride, and enthusiasm of the NAVO Survey Team and the Military Sealift Command crew. It was an absolute blast to get back in my summer whites and spend the evening visiting with old friends. The concern and support of our old "family" was a huge boost to our spirits.

The conference dinner was a luau. Ty scraped up a pair of the expensive tickets for Nancy and me. Actually, one of them was his. I guess going to a touristy hotel luau isn't a special night out if you live just up the hill. Unfortunately, rain forced us inside. But we did enjoy spending the evening with our New Orleans friends, Jim and Cynthia Bassich. Cynthia is a recent cancer survivor who coached me through much of my ordeal. We laughed about flying 6,000 miles to finally get together for an evening when we had a hard time coordinating our schedules for an evening together back in Louisiana. Toward the end of the luau, I hit the limit of my daily endurance. I enjoyed the professional Polynesian dancers, but when they started to drag audience members to the stage, I was more than ready to go. Believe me, there are a lot better things in the world than watching engineers do the hula.

◆   ◆   ◆

Traveling by air in the last months of 2001 was eye opening. Al-Qaeda's attack against the World Trade Center towers may have been much more dramatic and more successful than they had ever hoped on September 11th, but the lasting impact was not close to what they expected. Instead of instigating a widespread Islamic uprising against the West, they turned the opinion of most of the world against their cause. Allied military operations soon dealt a severe blow to their infrastructure and organization in Afghanistan. Nevertheless, the al-Qaeda goal of western economic disruption was successful to some degree, especially in the airline industry. The airlines operate on a relatively thin profit margin in the best of times. In 2001 they were already dealing with a recession when they were jolted by the terrorist attacks.

By the time we left for Hawaii, all of our flight times had changed in the airline schedule shifts and contractions. Our resulting itinerary had us leave New Orleans earlier and get to Hawaii later. The return trip was the same—we started early and finished late. Of course, we followed the airline suggestions and arrived at our departure airport several hours before our scheduled takeoff time. The extra hours were spent passing time as comfortably as we could in airport terminals.

This would have been a good trip to belong to one of the fancy airline clubs. They have much nicer furniture than the USO.

Over the years, my Navy travels took me to several dozen different countries. The recruiting commercials didn't lie. I did see the world, and it was an adventure! I always wondered if Americans truly appreciated our precious freedoms and our generally carefree approach to life. Whenever I witnessed airport security measures in southern Europe, the Middle East, and the Pacific Rim, I always thought that Americans would never put up with the restrictions that were common elsewhere in the world. In 2001, we had no choice. I was pleased to see that most people could appreciate the wisdom of balancing freedom and security. Travelers were universally tired, but almost always patient.

In the coming decades, I suspect that Americans will continually debate where to strike the balance between liberty and safety. As discomforting as it is to people who have spent their lives under the mistaken belief that "it couldn't happen here," there is no way to 100% guarantee that terrorists will never again be able to attack our civilians. We must continually weigh the risks and decide what level is acceptable. Risk reduction costs money and freedom.

In my own way, along with the country in general, I went through a major rebalancing of personal risks with personal freedom in the autumn of 2001. Before cancer, I knew what was good for me when it came to reducing health risks, but I didn't always do what was best. As a surviving cancer warrior, I am no longer free to eat as much as I want of whatever I want, sleep too little, or enjoy the Gulf Coast sunshine without layering on the sunscreen. I still enjoy a Burger King Whopper and fries, but now I am much more inclined to get my fast food from Subway. Exercise is not optional—it is mandatory. Nobody legislated these new life rules for me. I wanted to reduce the risks, so I had to put restrictions on myself. It is worth it. It keeps you on the right side of the grass.

12

The Good Days

SITREP #16

11/20/01

Dear Family, Friends, Shipmates, Classmates, Argonauts, and IHMCers,

Happy Thanksgiving, everyone! The more I take the time to think about it, the more I realize how much I personally have for which to be thankful. Those who receive these SITREPs are, individually and collectively, at the top of my list. The love and support from family, friends, and colleagues has been an unexpected blessing this year.

I am especially thankful for the people at UWF's Institute for Human and Machine Cognition. I am back in my office at IHMC this week, working on Navy training issues. It's been nice to be back with all these friends for several hours a day. I find that I "hit the wall" by mid-afternoon. They are already letting me use an office, a computer, and phone. Do you think asking for a cot and sleeping bag would be too much?

Of course, I am also thankful for the fantastic progress in our country's war on terrorism and my own personal battles. According to Rear Admiral John Stufflebeem—my friend, classmate and Pentagon briefer extraordinaire—the Taliban and al-Qaeda have ceased to provide organized opposition. Now comes the hard part—finding and weeding out individual pockets of evil.

On the home front, the third cycle of chemo carpet-bombing is destroying any cancer cells that might have survived the initial onslaught. As I expected, this cycle was tougher than the previous two. It took a day or two longer to recuperate. Perhaps that's because the toxins have built up in my tissues as the treatment protocol progresses. Or possibly because I am so disgustingly out of shape. Or maybe because I had the seed of a cold when I started and as soon as the immune levels fell, it developed into a full-fledged cold. Ah well—half way there. To quote one of my favorite

20th century leaders, Sir Winston Churchill, "When you're going through hell, keep going."

GO USA! Larry

◆   ◆   ◆

"I've had good days and bad days and going-half-mad days" (from Jimmy Buffett's semi classic, *If the Phone Doesn't Ring, It's Me* on his 1984 *Last Mango in Paris* album.)

◆   ◆   ◆

In the middle of each chemo cycle I was rewarded with a handful of days where I felt absolutely wonderful. As the Dark Days ended and the side effects became more manageable, my mental outlook improved dramatically. Physically, I was a wreck—weak and tired with a stomach that was constantly messed up, but mentally I would enjoy a very pleasant high. All of a sudden, the sky was bluer, the music was prettier, and the jokes were funnier. I suppose the closest comparison I can make is to that magic period when you first fall in love.

I've always tried to enjoy life with a positive outlook, but the euphoric feeling between chemo treatments was unusual. Typically, I like to maintain an even emotional keel. I don't usually let setbacks get me too far down. I try to take lucky breaks and successes in stride. The chemo drugs changed the even keel to a roller coaster. After an unbelievably long four or five Dark Days of depression, my mood would shoot upward for an all-too-short four or five days of high spirits.

The good mood was fragile. If I got tired, it quickly evaporated. I learned to protect my happy days by mixing a little exercise, a lot of rest, and a few prayers of thanks. Without these good days, I'm not sure how I could have faced the next round of Dark Days. Each cycle, I tried to hold on to the *joie de vivre* as I approached the next round of drugs, but I couldn't. The knowledge of what was to come was enough to quash the best of moods.

The Chemo Calendar was kind to me when it came to the holidays. The Columbus Day weekend, our Hawaii trip, Thanksgiving, and Christmas all fell during the good days of their respective cycles. Only New Year's Eve was during the Dark Days. If I had to pick one holiday to miss, that would have been my choice. New Year's is my least favorite holiday of the year, anyway. I got up on January 1, 2002 with a headache, upset stomach, and a miserable hung over feeling—and I didn't even have to get dressed up the night before.

It took a couple of cycles before I recognized the depression-elation mood swing pattern and tied it to the chemo calendar. The first round of good days coincided with my release from the hospital and our road trip to Louisiana. At the time, I attributed my good mood to my new freedom. I had Nancy's cooking instead of the institutional food from the hospital kitchen. No one came into my bedroom in the middle of the night to check my vital signs, so I rested much better. I was able to get out and about—as much as the swollen foot and recovering ankle would allow.

After I turned in my crutches, Nancy and I made a trip to Pensacola Beach to watch the sunset one beautiful October afternoon. Since the Emerald Coast of the Florida Panhandle runs east and west, you can only see the sun set into the Gulf of Mexico during the winter half of the year. During the summer, when sunset is north of due west, it continues past the beach, over the hotels, and on over Pensacola Bay and the mainland. I tested my strength by walking to the end of the new Pensacola Beach fishing pier. At 400 yards out and then another slow 400 yards back to the beach end, it taxed me just about to the limit.

◆   ◆   ◆

I still don't know whether my good mood inspired the trip to the beach, or if I was subconsciously trying to extend the happy days. In each of the later cycles, I intentionally made a trip to the beach during the period of high spirits. Once I figured out that the feeling was of limited duration, I nurtured it to try to extend it as long as possible. By driving over the toll bridge to the beach, I took a mini-vacation from life in the apartment. Parking my car in the shadow of our wonderfully tacky beach ball-painted water tower, I enjoyed the smells, sounds, and sights of one of the absolutely prettiest white sand beaches in the world.

I have always enjoyed the beach. My parents love it. As a kid, the highlight of our year was when we loaded up the station wagon and made our weeklong trip to Wildwood, NJ every August. After their sons grew up, Mom and Dad left the hectic beach resort scene behind by taking their time at the shore on little Chincoteague Island on the northernmost coast of Virginia. Unless you are there during the annual Pony Penning festivities in the last week of July, Chincoteague is quiet and peaceful. Of course, when Jim and Lindsay were young, they wanted to see the ponies swim across the sound from Assateague. Mom and Dad fought the crowds. That's what grandparents are for!

My children are wonderfully lucky. In addition to my parents' little beach house in Chincoteague, they've enjoyed trips to North Carolina's Outer Banks almost every year of their lives. When we were stationed in Norfolk in 1981, the year Jim was born, we took Nancy's parents on a day-trip down the coast. We stopped at the office of one of the earliest timeshare vacation places to listen to the sales pitch and get a gift certificate for free dinners. At least, I was just planning on getting a free dinner. Instead, we ended up with a family reunion on the Outer Banks every June. With a growing family of grandchildren, Jack and Kitty decided that owning a few weeks of vacation timeshares would be an excellent way to travel and still enjoy time at the shore with their extended family. They now own eight weeks each year of timeshare vacations. In addition to our June beach party, Mom and Dad Ludwick have treated their children and grandchildren to Disney World, Hawaii, ski resort weeks, New Orleans, and Europe.

But the beach is still my first choice. I was a Jacques Costeau ocean-ographer. It really isn't surprising that many of my colleagues in Navy METOC grew up watching the Costeau television specials and the Lloyd Bridges television series, *Sea Hunt*. I went off to the Naval Academy with an existing strong affection for the sea. It wasn't until I made my first voyage across the Atlantic on Youngster Cruise that I found out that what I really love about the sea is where it meets the shore! Once you're out of sight of land, the scenery gets pretty boring. Besides, in my day, when women didn't sail on Navy ships, I never saw a bikini beyond the limits of the Exclusive Economic Zone. The ocean is nice, but you need to put it next to a stretch of warm, soft sand to really appreciate it.

◆   ◆   ◆

The second round of good days took us to Hawaii. Again, I attributed my good mood to the anticipation of our long-planned trip to see great friends during our week in paradise. After the terrific, but physically taxing week, I crashed hard when we returned to the mainland. We got home on Saturday and drove to Pensacola Sunday to begin Cycle #3. During the long trip home, I picked up a cold bug. As soon as the immune system started to weaken as the blood counts fell, it became a full-fledged cold. Mentally, I was down, and physically I was weaker than ever. The toxins were building up in my tissues. Plus, I wasn't even half way through the chemo treatments. During the Dark Days I wasn't sure how I was going to make it through three more cycles. The recovery from cycle #3 took two days longer than any of the other rounds, either before or after.

When my mood recovered after that cycle, it was Thanksgiving week. I had to have a complete blood count on Wednesday before driving with Lindsay to Louisiana. Leaving the offices of Hematology and Oncology Associates at the Sacred Heart Hospital, I got on the elevator with one of the pleasant hospital workers in the purple scrubs.

She took a look at my peach fuzz hair and said, "We have a **lot** to be thankful for, don't we?"

I was emphatic, "We **sure** do!"

She introduced herself as a breast cancer survivor. Once you're in the cancer family, you never leave.

SITREP #17

12/3/01

Dear Family, Friends, Shipmates, Classmates, Argonauts, and IHMCers,

When you get to the mid-point of a Navy deployment, it's known as "hump day." After that day, you're over-the-hump and looking forward to returning to homeport. Today is hump day in the chemotherapy cruise. It's the first day of Cycle #4. My blood counts show that the chemicals are doing the expected—and weakening my immune system as a side effect. The good news is that I've recovered so well that Dr. Tan decided to increase the dosage of carboplatin. When the nurse mixed up the prescription and hooked me up this afternoon, she said, "Wow, you're getting a big dose!" Colin Powell recommends that if you're going, go with overwhelming force!

We had a very nice Thanksgiving with Jim and Lindsay both home from college. We did a lot of eating, a lot of laundry, and got a good start on Christmas decorations over the weekend. Lindsay caught up with all her high school friends who were back in Mandeville for the first time. Jim mostly caught up on sleep. After we all returned to our various schools, Nancy finished decorating the house. It looks great. To get fired up for cycle 4, we went to Ingrid and Fred Zeile's annual Army-Navy party. Army won, but Nancy and I each won a quarter of the pool, so the game wasn't a total loss.

We've found that spending time with friends and family inspires us and keeps our spirits high. Thanks to all of you—whether you live close by and we see you in person, or if you live far away and we "spend time with you" electronically.

GO USA! Larry

13

Winston, Jimmy, and Garth

SITREP #18

12/21/01

Dear Family, Friends, Shipmates, Classmates, Argonauts, and IHMCers,

Happy Holidays and Merry Christmas to you all! For those of you with whom we usually exchange Christmas cards…please don't think we've forgotten you. Nurse Nancy is working on them as I write.

As my life is temporarily under the control of the chemo calendar, it looks like Christmas Day will be a great day to eat, drink, and be merry. Cycle #5 will be the week between Christmas and New Year's. (I get to suffer with a New Year's Day hangover, and I don't even have to get dressed up the night before!) Guess I'll just lie on the couch and watch football. Yes, I know that's what I'd be doing anyway! But now I have an excuse.

The good news is that the sixth and LAST chemo cycle will be finished by the end of January. Hallelujah! I'll say goodbye to Osama the IV stand forever. Maybe our troops and allies will bid a not-so-fond farewell to the really evil Osama before then. If not then…well, as long as it takes, Baby!

Earlier this week, the Jimmy V Foundation's annual basketball fundraiser was held at the Meadowlands Arena. ESPN replayed the speech that former North Carolina State basketball coach Jim Valvano gave shortly before his death from cancer in 1993. Jimmy encouraged all of us to do three things every day—

- *Laugh.*
- *Think.*
- *Be emotional.*

I think that's good advice. Couple it with Jimmy V's motto—"NEVER GIVE UP. DON'T EVER GIVE UP!"

GO USA! Larry

I have always been inclined to live my life by bumper sticker philosophies. I don't know if it is a sign of a short attention span or a lack of concentration, but I prefer short, pithy sayings that summarize more complex and meaningful strategies. The advice of Winston Churchill stuck in my mind throughout the chemo months.

"If you're going through hell, keep going."

Churchill is one of my heroes. He was not a particularly wonderful human being. He was brusque, inconsiderate, commanding, intolerant, and overwhelming. Yet he was the perfect wartime prime minister. He inspired the people of Great Britain to hold on against Hitler when the rest of the countries of the western world were either defeated or not yet ready to join the fight. More than sixty years later, his stirring quotes still make great bumper sticker philosophies.

During the *joie de vivre* times of each cycle, not only were the sky bluer and the jokes funnier, the quotes I read and heard seemed more meaningful than they ever did before. When Lindsay and I drove from Pensacola to Mandeville on the day before Thanksgiving, we played a Garth Brooks CD. A line from one song struck me as a good bumper sticker for my cancer experience.

"I could have missed the pain, but I would have had to miss the dance."

By the mid-point of chemotherapy, I was starting to believe that maybe I was going to come out the other end as one of the truly lucky ones. I surely would have liked to skip the pain of the surgeries and the misery of chemo, but the rewards looked promising. I definitely did not want to miss the dance.

Another recent country music hit, Lee Ann Womack's *"I Hope You Dance,"* was an inspiration for me when Nancy and I decided to leave the Navy and start our new life on the Emerald Coast. Womack sings, "I hope you still feel small when you stand beside the ocean. Whenever one door closes, I hope one more opens. Promise me that you'll give faith a fighting chance. And when you get the chance to sit it out or dance...I hope you dance."

◆   ◆   ◆

In 1993, Jimmy Valvano knew that his dance would not last much longer. Famous for his exuberant personality while leading the NC State Wolfpack basketball team, he used his fame to shine a bright light on cancer. In his heart, he knew that new research was not going to find answers in time to save him. Nevertheless, he campaigned to the very end of his life to raise cancer research funds. The Jimmy V Foundation is one of the leading contributors of money to promising new therapies, drugs, and treatment protocols. For all I know, Jimmy could have helped save my life.

Even before cancer became my personal enemy—back in the days when I thought of it as a terrible disease that only happened to other people—Jimmy's speech on ESPN made me laugh and cry. When I saw the replay during the 2001 tournament, I took his words to heart.

> "To me there are three things everyone should do every day. Number one is laugh. You should laugh every day. Number two is think—spend some time in thought. Number three, you should have your emotions move you to tears. If you laugh, think, and cry, that's a heck of a day.
>
> Ralph Waldo Emerson said, 'Nothing great was ever achieved without enthusiasm.' I urge all of you to enjoy your life; to be enthusiastic every day; to keep your dreams alive in spite of your problems.
>
> Now I look where I am and what I want to do. With ESPN's support, we are starting the Jimmy V Foundation for cancer

research. Its motto is **_Don't Give Up. Don't ever give up._** That's what I'm going to try to do every minute I have left. I will thank God for the day and the moment I have. I know I gotta go. But I have one last thing to say. Cancer can take all my physical abilities. It cannot touch my mind, it cannot touch my heart and it cannot touch my soul. And those three things are going to carry on forever."

Enthusiasm is vital! It was my secret weapon in my war. I discovered an inner zeal for life. I didn't want to simply survive cancer. I wanted to kick its butt! I always try to bring enthusiasm to every thing I do. I find that people will forgive mistakes and errors if they know you really care about what you are trying to do. As a coach, I don't mind errors made by players who are aggressive. As a leader, I can easily forgive mistakes made by someone who is **doing something**. I have no use for people who sit around, afraid to act, in fear of making a mistake.

◆   ◆   ◆

A generation before Churchill, Theodore Roosevelt was a leader with passion and enthusiasm. I've kept this quote on my desk for many years. It may be a bit long to put on a bumper sticker, but it is one I try to live by.

"It is not the critic who counts; not the man who points out how the strong man stumbled, or where the doer of deeds could have done them better. The credit belongs to the man who is actually in the arena, whose face is marred by dust and sweat and blood; who strives valiantly; who errs and comes short again and again; who knows the great enthusiasms, the great devotions; who spends himself in a worthy cause; who at the best, knows in the end the triumph of high achievement, and who, at the worst, if he fails, at least fails while daring greatly, so that his place shall never be with those timid souls who know neither victory or defeat."

I drew strength and inspiration from many other bumper-sticker philosophies during the cancer journey. Some I read in books or magazines. Some came from e-mails. Some only stuck in my mind for a day or two. I didn't write any of them down. I can only include the ones that made a lasting impression and remain in my long-term memory.

"I have cancer, but cancer doesn't have me!"

I wish I could claim that I made that one up by myself. It exactly captures the way I felt during the battle. It was the way I wanted the world to see me. It was the feeling I tried to convey in each SITREP.

"Pain is temporary. Quitting is forever."

Lance Armstrong is an expert on pain. Elite cyclists endure pain that would make the normal person quit on the first hill. Lance applied the lessons he had absorbed during his cycling career to his cancer recovery. Early on, when the pain of the surgeries brought tears to my eyes, I just kept repeating, "Pain is temporary. Pain is temporary." Quitting was **never** an option.

"Pray like everything depends on God and fight like everything depends on you."

Our friends run the full gamut of religious belief. Many are convinced that God, the Great Physician, healed me personally. Others would rather put their faith in medicine and discount the value of prayer. I find myself with a foot firmly in each camp, and a strong belief in both possibilities. Frankly, I don't care what cured me, but I think that a combination of science and religion is a powerful weapon. I believe doctors and researchers can do wonderful things with the science of medicine. I consider this manmade medical care the "natural" cure. But I have no doubt that there is a greater power. This "super" power guides the scientists in their work. I'm convinced that the super power will answer every cancer warrior's prayers for strength, courage, patience, and hope. When you put the two forces together, you get the "supernatural." That's the team you want working for your cure!

"Let's roll!"

Todd Beamer's last words ring out as the battle cry of the War on Terrorism. He and his fellow passengers took on the hijackers over Pennsylvania in the first American offensive reaction of the war. They prevented one team of terrorists from accomplishing their mission. I wonder if I would have had the same courage had I been on the plane instead of in a hospital bed. I'll never know. But I do know those passengers who refused to die quietly are heroes for all of us.

"God Bless America and Let's Play Ball!"

After 9/11, Bruce Desporte began closing his e-mails with this phrase. I adopted it right away as the title of my softball chapter. I kept it in mind in the Dark Days as I tried to mentally transport myself to the coming softball season. I repeated it to myself as I worked out to get back in shape. Now whenever I have a home plate umpire assignment, I use it proudly to start the game. It is the only time I have ever gotten a cheer as an umpire.

◆   ◆   ◆

As I said, I think I must have a limited attention span. I enjoyed a whole shelf full of books during my recuperation from surgery and during my energy-limited days as a couch potato. But the two that made the biggest impact were two of the shortest books to make the New York Times bestseller list during the last decade of the 20th Century. The books are completely different, and each impressed me in a totally different way.

When I first read Spencer Johnson's *Who Moved My Cheese?* I thought it was a trivial piece of make believe. It is a fable about change and how we adapt to it. Four characters—two mice, and two mouse-sized people—live in a big maze. Every day they go to a specific place in the maze to feed on the supply of cheese that they know will be there. One day, the cheese is gone. The two mice, Sniff and Scurry, immediately head off in search of a new source of cheese. The little humans, Hem and Haw, have a much harder time adapting to change. Haw gradually learns the lessons of change and eventually finds an even better feeding station, but Hem refuses to accept that his cheese has been moved.

The author encourages his readers to figure out which character best describes them. Sniff is constantly looking for change and is ready to head off in another direction. Scurry reacts to change by running quickly through the maze until he finds a new situation he likes. Hem never adapts and suffers for his rigid adherence to a routine that no longer works for him. Haw slowly learns the lessons and forces himself to adapt to the change that has been forced upon him when his cheese was moved.

I blew off this book as a bit of a waste of time. I could see how it could be a useful exercise if you are leading a seminar on change, but I thought it too simplistic. It didn't even give me any good bumper sticker philosophies, despite the fact that Haw regularly found key thoughts written on the walls of the maze. But ever since I read it, Dr. Johnson's lessons keep coming back to me. Even small alterations to my plans trigger the thought, "They moved my cheese!" (By the way, I identify with Scurry. I don't typically seek out change, but I'm quick to accept it and run off to look for a new way to get the job done.)

◆   ◆   ◆

The other book that hit hard was Mitch Albom's tribute to his dying college professor, *Tuesdays with Morrie*. I had very little in common with Morrie Schwartz. He was a small, Jewish, very liberal professor of Sociology at an upper-crust private college in New England. Morrie contracted Amyotrophic Lateral Sclerosis—ALS, or Lou Gehrig's Disease. He knew it would kill him. There is not yet a cure, and ALS is always fatal. Mitch Albom was a favorite student of Morrie's two decades before the end. When he heard about his old teacher's disease, he returned for a visit. Together, they decided to work on one last paper. Albom flew in from Detroit every Tuesday so he could write the story of Morrie's final battle.

I was different from Morrie Schwartz in every aspect I can think of—from physical size to family background to politics. His disease was certain to kill him. Mine was a serious threat, but I steadfastly refused to even consider that it would kill me. Still, I found that Morrie's approach to death is a lesson in how every one of the rest of us can live.

Morrie Schwartz believed that once you know how to die, then you really know how to live. He thought he could help bridge the gap by making his own death a lesson in living. His humor, compassion, and courage in his last six month's of life inspired me through an entire cycle of Dark Days.

Morrie adopted a Buddhist tactic that I in turn borrowed from him. Every day I imagine a little bird on my shoulder. Each day I ask the bird if today is my last day of this life. Because we don't know, do we? In our culture, we tend to believe and act as if we are indestructible. Even people in dangerous professions think it "won't happen to me." The men and women of our armed forces, our police and firefighters, and even airline passengers are undoubtedly more aware of the fragility of life than the average American. But they certainly don't expect to die. The terrorist victims surely didn't think they were entering the Trade Center towers or the Pentagon for the last time. Given another chance, would they have done things differently before leaving home that morning? Probably.

"Is today the day, little bird?"

Morrie Schwartz allowed himself a little self-pity. He mourned his failing body as he said goodbye to his family, friends, and associates. He cried for himself if he felt like it. Then he got on with the business of getting the most out of every day. He lived each day as if it were his last, even though he knew almost exactly when the last one was scheduled.

I honestly didn't spend much time mourning my condition. I figured it was a waste of precious mental energy. In some moments of weakness, I did feel sorry for myself. I kept thinking that it just was not fair that I had been drafted into the cancer war. As I got to know Morrie Schwartz through his favorite student's last assignment, I thought it was so unfair that such a wonderful, gentle soul should have to suffer so much. It made me recall one of my favorite (and my children's least favorite) bumper sticker philosophies,

"Life's Not Fair!"

I suspect every father in the world has used this line when his child whines, "Daaa-aad, that's not fair!"

"Sorry kid, but life's not fair."

If you are a baby boomer, you might remember the old Parker Brothers' Game of Life. You got a little plastic car and little blue and pink pegs as you went around the board according to the number that came up on the spinner. It was a pretty fair game. In fact, the rules were printed right on the inside of the box cover! In the real Game of Life, however, it's different. In the real game:

- Life's not fair.
- It takes slightly longer than one lifetime to play.
- You have to start playing before you know you're in the game.
- The playing field isn't level.
- Some people get to play by different rules.
- Once you figure out the rules, they change.
- You don't get a mulligan.

BUT! *(And this is the **real** power hidden under this bumper sticker)*...In the real Game of Life, you have one HUGE advantage. You get to keep your own score. And you get to set up the scoring system as it suits you and your God. In the end—that's the only score that counts.

Allow me to suggest a few scoring categories you should make worth "triple points" as you play your own game of life.

- Family,

- Keeping yourself in good physical condition,

- Having fun at your job, and

- Giving something back to your community.

Life may not be fair. But life sure is good!

14

Eat Less and Move Around More

SITREP #19

1/14/02

Dear Family, Friends, Shipmates, Classmates, Argonauts, and IHMCers,

OK, OK. Back by popular demand...Situation Report #19. The lovely Nurse Nancy says she's fielded too many phone calls and e-mails from friends wondering how things are going. I apologize for causing concern. In this case, no news is good news. The war continues according to our strategic plan.

Chemo cycle five was December 27-29. Christmas was wonderful—New Year's was not-so-wonderful. The last chemo period is scheduled for next week...January 21, 22, and 23. Four weeks later we'll begin a series of tests and scans to see if there is any evidence of cancer anywhere.

I suppose I do have a bit of news to report. I've been able to begin exercising again. The surgery and chemo fatigue had me on the sidelines for over three months. Now I walk a mile four days a week. That isn't much, but since I finish out of breath and my muscles ache, I classify it as a moderately strenuous workout! The last chemo cycle will put me out of the game for another week or ten days, but from that point on I should be able to make steady progress. (Unless I do something stupid, like try to do too much too soon.) My goal is to be in shape to umpire by the time summer softball starts.

I wish you all a happy and healthy 2002. Do one thing for me, will you? Make a resolution to use liberal amounts of sunscreen this year (even if you never burn).

GO USA! Larry

When I saw the extent of the original surgery on my ankle on 9/11, I was shocked. Within hours, the horror of the terrorist attacks made that first shock of the day seem minor. As I watched the news, I gradually recovered my bearings. Then I started wondering how my life and exercise routines would have to change to accommodate my new condition.

At first, I didn't comprehend that Dr. Schneider had managed to remove all the cancerous tissue without removing any muscle or critical ligaments or structural elements. The hole in my leg looked so huge that it seemed to me that my leg and ankle must have been severely damaged.

The muscles may have been intact, but the lymph system was severely interrupted. My foot was swollen all the time. It really ballooned if I didn't keep it elevated. The swelling concerned me more than anything during the first month of my war. Even the cancer itself didn't worry me as much as the swollen leg and foot. I understood the battle ahead of me to beat the cancer. The survival odds based on existing case histories of Merkle Cell weren't good, but at least we had an aggressive plan of attack. The potential extent of the swelling problem, on the other hand, was an unknown.

In the first few weeks, I was disappointed that neither Dr. Schneider nor Dr. Tan could reassure me that the swelling would ever be under control. Perhaps too much of the lower leg lymph system was gone. They were also considering whether I would need radiation treatments to the lower leg or to the remaining lymph nodes in the groin. Radiation to either area would significantly complicate the swelling problem. I visualized years of wearing special compression stockings and wraps. Several times I told Nancy that if the swelling kept me from walking and exercising, they could just amputate the whole foot and I would learn to walk and work out using a prosthesis.

◆   ◆   ◆

I knew I needed exercise. I wanted to exercise. But my ability to exercise was greatly limited for months. For the first month, I was not allowed to put any weight at all on my right leg. For two weeks, the surgical wound was open. Then the skin graft needed time to adhere to the underlying tissue. Early on, I actually enjoyed the physical challenge of moving about on crutches. It gave me a chance to successfully do something with the body that had seemed to betray me in other ways. Once I was unhooked from Osama the IV stand, I took my crutch workout into the wide passageways of the Naval Hospital. First the nurses' station was the goal, then the elevators.

When I put the crutches away, the weakness of the ankle restricted my walk to a slow and painful hobble. Even though it marked good progress, the hobble was not nearly so physically or mentally rewarding as flying around on crutches. Of course, none of my forms of locomotion—the crutches, the cane, nor the hobbling—was conducive to any type of real aerobic exercise. Even as the ankle healed and the skin graft took hold, my overall physical condition rapidly grew flabbier and weaker. About the time I gained reliable use of the ankle and leg, the chemotherapy calendar induced a weariness that made a brisk walk absolutely unthinkable.

Out of necessity, I was able to maintain at least one of my regular exercise habits throughout my cancer journey. Every couple of days I stretched my lower back, did crunches, back strengtheners, and a light abdominal workout. Even in the hospital bed, I did these as best I could. I knew from long experience that more than three days without doing this exercise set would leave me with considerable pain and stiffness in the lower back.

Each day I had to balance my desire for physical activity with the need to manage the swelling. For the first few weeks after I started putting weight on my foot, I lived in a pair of rubber slide-on sandals. I adjusted the velcro strap on the right shoe to something far beyond EEE width. That worked fine in October, but with cooler weather and our trip to Hawaii coming up, I needed to find a way to get my foot into a real shoe.

New Balance cross-trainers were the answer. I wasn't using them for workouts, but they got plenty of use during my inactive months, nonetheless. I loosened the laces of the right sneaker as far as they would go, put it on, and then cinched it up snug. It turned out to be a good compression shoe. By tightening the laces, the excess fluid in the foot was forced upward. I really believe the continued pressure helped encourage the generation of new lymph circulation pathways to bypass the missing ankle tissue.

◆   ◆   ◆

In Hawaii, it is customary to remove your shoes when you enter someone's home. I guess that's partly due to the strong Oriental influence in the islands. Plus, nobody wants the famous Hawaiian red dirt tracked onto their rugs. Maybe that's why at least half the population considers flip-flops to be formal footwear. They're easily removed on the way in, and you don't even slow down as you step into them on the way out.

I took my cross-trainers off at the Aldingers' door on the first two days of our visit and enjoyed walking around barefoot. But without the constricting support, my foot swelled too much and too quickly. I had to keep the swelling down so I could wear my white dress shoes with my uniform for Ty's retirement. I returned to a tightly laced shoe whenever I was out of bed. I'm genuinely anticipating our next trip to Hawaii. It's going to be sandals and bare feet for me!

Not surprisingly, the red-eye flight back from Hawaii, with airport delays on both ends and a long layover when we switched planes in the middle, resulted in the most troublesome swelling of the whole war. We were out of bed for more than thirty hours. I propped my foot on our carry-on luggage as we waited, but it did little good. By the time we got home, my leg was swollen from knee to the top of the sneaker. Even full-cut khaki trousers were tight over the calf.

◆   ◆   ◆

Five days later I completely stopped worrying about swelling. When chemo cycle #3 put me in bed for the Dark Days, the swelling immediately went down. I knew then that it would be manageable in the future. Using the tightly-laced shoe kept the foot from swelling, and my body had established a good enough system to reduce the leg swelling, provided I was patient enough to give it time. Plus, at my cycle #3 examination, Dr. Tan told me that radiation would not be necessary. I suspect that I will have to manage some minor swelling for years, but that's a small price to pay for full mobility.

My desire for exercise wasn't just a physical feeling. It was a mental necessity. I find that if I don't exercise regularly, it impacts my mood. Micki Zorn, my secretary at NAVO would tell me, "You're getting cranky. You better go work out."

We had a deal. She put a ninety-minute block of time on my calendar every day to go to the Stennis Space Center Wellness Center. I told her she could move it around, but not to delete it without my permission. Many times she moved it to 6:30 am, but I almost always squeezed in a workout if I wasn't traveling. Even on the road, I tried to get to the hotel exercise room every day for a quick stretch and light workout.

◆   ◆   ◆

The Wellness Center staff and I used to laugh about the crazy radio weight-loss commercials that aired seemingly constantly every day. We shared a distrust of the fad diets that other members of the center tried from time to time. Dr. Adkin's, Sugar Busters, cabbage soup, Metabolife, and even phen-fen had proponents among our friends. I suppose that there is fairly solid science behind some of these diet plans. I know that diet books certainly make up a lucrative segment in the publishing business.

There certainly is a need in the United States for effective weight-loss strategies. Obesity is an "epidemic" that costs us more every year. Our social advances have put us in a position that nearly everyone in the country has more than enough to eat. Our jobs have moved from physical work that burned lots of calories to mental tasks that we accomplish while sitting in padded chairs in air-conditioned comfort. We are eating more calories and burning fewer. We don't need gimmick diets. We need to change our lifestyles.

Scott, Anne, and I joked about writing our own diet book. But we decided it would never sell, since we didn't have a magical gimmick to allow our readers to "lose weight without exercise while eating as much as you want." Besides, our plan was far too short for a book. No matter how you look at weight loss programs, they all boil down to the same thing—***Eat Less and Move Around More.***

◆   ◆   ◆

I was in sorry shape by the time I could begin even minimal workouts. At the end of the Dark Days of each chemo cycle, I would feel like exercising again. In fact, it was the first sign that the chemical-induced depression was over. Now, when I say "exercise," I don't mean an hour at the gym. Actually, my first workout after each cycle usually consisted of walking down the three flights of stairs to the newspaper box, then using the stairs instead of the elevator to get back to our top-floor apartment. By the time I got back to the fourth floor I had to stop and rest with my hands on my knees to catch my breath.

Those three flights of stairs became my fitness marker. Before cancer, I often worked out on the back stairwells of high-rise hotels when I traveled on business. Most hotel fitness centers leave much to be desired, but a set of stairs is reliable. I used to jog-walk up and down the staircase until I reached as many as 120 floors. When I resumed exercise after surgery, I could just barely make it to the top of three flights. Gradually my wind got better until I could go from the parking lot to the apartment without stopping. By a month after the last chemo cycle, I wasn't even breathing too hard.

I gained almost ten pounds during the five months after surgery. Even more damning were the several pounds of muscle that had degenerated into fat during my days as a sofa-slug. I knew that resuming a regular exercise routine was vital to my mental health, my immune system, and my general physical well being.

At first, no one who saw me could possibly guess that I was exercising. I started making the four-minute walk to and from the Cognition Institute. Then I added short lunchtime walks through the Seville Quarter historical district, or (if the weather was particularly nice) along Pensacola Bay. My pace was slow and my distance was short. But I would find myself out of breath at the end of the walk. My muscles would become pleasantly stiff and sore. I knew I was doing more than beating cancer. I was on my way to becoming physically active again. It was a huge spirit-lifter.

By exercising in beautiful surroundings, I maximized the mental value of my physical workouts. During each of my trips to the beach, I took a walk along the Gulf of Mexico. I figured the soft and uneven sand was a great challenge to my ankle strength and stability. Besides, there's just something about dumping sand out of your shoes that makes you feel like you're on vacation! Walking on Pensacola Beach has other advantages. Even during the cooler months the "eyeball liberty" is pretty good, provided you choose a nice warm, sunny day.

If you tire of spotting bikini-clad spring breakers, there is always wildlife in abundance. Brown pelicans are almost as easily spotted as gulls. Shore birds hunt along the edge of the water. Twice I witnessed feeding frenzies as predators chased big schools of baitfish into the shallows.

One time a raft of more than a hundred sea-going ducks swam together parallel to the shore. They were all headed west into the setting sun, paddling along just inside the line where the waves began to break. Each time a wave threatened, each duck would dive under it like a body surfer. The hunting must have been especially good in the break zone, because the ducks certainly expended a lot of energy avoiding waves when they could have easily floated over them by moving just ten yards farther seaward. Individual ducks spent no more than three or four seconds swimming along before diving under the next wave and popping back to the surface. I laughed out loud at their antics.

After I got stronger, I began to take all of my lunchtime walks along Pensacola Bay. The traffic and stoplights made walking through the historic district too choppy, but the walk along the water was uninterrupted. Plus, the Hawkshaw Lagoon is home to more wildlife that I could enjoy during the workout. Herons, egrets, pelicans, and turtles were their every day. I kept an eye on the sky for ospreys that fished the bay. For most of the month of February, a kingfisher commandeered a dead tree branch to use as he stood the day shift lookout watch. In April a striking pair of Baltimore orioles moved in.

If you get tired of natural wonders, there are always man-made sights to see. Nearly every day during the winter months you could spot another common Florida migratory species, either at the beach or in town. The white-tufted, pot-bellied snowbirds are usually good for a chuckle. Who dresses these people?

After I finished the last chemo cycle, I increased my daily walks to two miles. I went outbound for a mile. It always took right around fifteen minutes. I measured my progress by timing how long it took me to walk the mile back to the office. On my first two-mile day, the return trip took more than twenty minutes! When I am in decent shape, it should be easy for me to walk the return mile in a quicker time than my first mile. The first couple of minutes of the outbound walk are slow, since I have to warm up my aching knees before pushing too hard. Until I get a few blocks away from the office, I feel like the

Tin Man before Dorothy found his oilcan. Finally, seven weeks into my exercise program, on the first day of spring, I made the trip back to the office in less than fifteen minutes. A strong wind at my back probably made the difference, but I took credit, wind-aided or not!

◆   ◆   ◆

After the skin graft, my ankle rarely hurt, unless I was on my feet for too long at a stretch. As the months went on, I could stand and walk for longer and longer periods. While I was never in real pain, there was always a sensation in the grafted area. It felt a bit like your hands feel if you touch your thumbs and fingertips of both hands together and then push to stretch your hands as far as possible. During the first months after the skin graft, some of the nerves regenerated in the new tissue. Often the synapses would fire unexpectedly when a new connection was made. It felt like small electrical shocks. It was surprising, but not unpleasant, especially since I knew it meant that the tissue was alive and healing.

Toward the end of the chemotherapy regimen, my ankle finally recovered sufficiently to start physical therapy. The open holes in the skin graft had continued to heal slowly, even though the chemo wiped out most of the immune and repair functions that would normally have been available. In all, I had to wear the gauze and Ace bandage dressings on my ankle for more than 270 consecutive days.

The physical therapist removed the dressing and examined the wound carefully. He had me stand, bend, and walk up and down the hall as he knelt and scrutinized my ankle. In the end, he decided against any strenuous therapy program, since the remaining holes were right where the skin flexed the most. He felt that moderate walking was OK, but that anything else would further delay healing. I was disappointed, because I secretly wanted to be pushed hard. I was prepared for the classic physical therapy "no pain—no gain" approach. Instead, he told me to exercise patience. Once again I was advised to practice patience. I practiced, but I still didn't get the hang of it. Reminds me of the old story about the mother who overheard her teenager in prayer:

"Lord, please grant me patience. And I WANT IT RIGHT NOW!"

The therapist commented on my lack of flexibility. I know all too well that flexibility is the third part of a good fitness program, along with strength and aerobic capacity. I knew the importance of stretching, and I even knew how to stretch. I just never took the time to do it right. From surgery until that first PT appointment, I had pretty much quit stretching altogether. My generally poor flexibility became appalling. I think the therapist's exact quote was, "Captain, you can't even spell 'stretch,' can you?"

Fifteen minutes of stretching twice a day was the prescription. It allowed me to experience a little of the pain for which I had mentally prepared. It helped. I still suffer from a limited range of motion, but I'm much better off than I was, even before cancer.

The PT folks also gave me a Styrofoam half-cylinder to help me work on my balance and the strength and flexibility of the small muscles around the ankle and foot. I stood on one foot on the cylinder, round side down, for 30–45 seconds at a time. It helped a lot. Eventually, I got to the point that I could keep my balance with my eyes closed.

At the beginning of the PT session I had to fill out a form. One of the questions was, "What do you expect to gain from therapy?" My answer was that I wanted to be able to resume umpiring as soon as possible. As he summed up our first session, the therapist said he couldn't recommend umpiring.

"Because of my ankle?"

"No, because your knees are so bad!"

Well, I've umpired on achy knees for years. It may not be the best thing for me, but I'm not about to quit.

In fact, I accelerated my original schedule for my umpiring come back. I had originally hoped to be ready by the end of May, in time for the summer fastpitch season. But the Northwest Florida Umpire Association held a clinic as I was hitting the joyous days after the final chemo cycle at the end of January. I went, and in my exuberance, I signed up to call games during UWF's month of Spring Fling tournaments. If I needed any more inspiration to get into decent aerobic condition, stabilize the ankle, improve flexibility, and strengthen my legs, this was it. The last thing I wanted to do was look like a lazy umpire by not being able to hustle when I was on the field.

I can't remember a much more satisfying feeling than the evening after I called my first three games of college softball. I was behind the plate for two of them. When Nancy called, I was sitting on the sofa in the apartment, with my sore toe in a bucket of hot water, ice bags on both knees, and a beer in my hand. Sure was good to be back to normal!

15

The New Normal

SITREP #20

1/28/02

Dear Family, Friends, Shipmates, Classmates, Argonauts, and IHMCers,

It has been quite an eventful ten days for Nancy and me. Chemotherapy ended. The Mandeville Magic Box closed its doors. My medical paperwork went off to Washington. We accepted an offer on our house in Louisiana and we made an offer on a house in Florida. Plus, the washing machine we've had for our entire marriage expired—after about 12,000 loads. I think it must be time for us to really, actually, finally get on with our new life.

To me, the end of chemo is far and away the highlight of all of these milestones. After all, we've bought houses and appliances before. I suspect that a few months down the road my mind will bury the chemo memories. I certainly hope they get buried deeply and permanently. This is one of those things about which you "never say never," but I certainly don't wish to spend any more time in the oncologist's recliner chairs. Hopefully, I am now clawing my way back toward normal again. The only trouble is that I'm not exactly sure that I'll recognize "normal" when I get there.

Before she became the Lovely Nurse Nancy, Nancy spent more than three years as one of the Magic Box's part time toy experts. The owners decided to consolidate operations in their New Orleans store. Some of the Northshore staff will move to a newly opened Mandeville toy store, but Nancy's days there will depend on our actual move date.

Both of our real estate contracts are "contingent." That is, we won't close on our new home until we sell the Louisiana house. That won't happen until our buyers can sell their house. I don't know how far back this home selling daisy chain extends. Maybe someone has to sell a house trailer in Oklahoma so everyone can move on.

GO USA! Larry

After surviving surgeries, radiation, chemotherapy, and months of seemingly endless testing, injections, blood counts, and worry, you would think that cancer warriors would welcome the opportunity to put cancer behind them and just get on with life. It is easier said than done, I assure you. Like it or not, life has changed, and you can't go back to the normal life you once knew.

Cynthia Bassich is about a year ahead of me in the cancer war. With her recent experience, I was always anxious to compare notes with her throughout my journey. She pointed out to me that what we considered a normal life before cancer is now part of our past. Cyn sent me some wise advice in response to SITREP #20.

"I know what you mean by saying you hope that you will recognize 'normal' when you get there. I'm not sure I have recognized 'normal.' I'm not sure that 'normal' ever is the same as it once was. Things return to a normalcy, but I'm not sure they are ever really the same as they were before such a life-changing event. I don't necessarily think that this is a bad thing. I think that we are changed forever for the better in the long run. We know now who we truly are, 'what we are made of,' and we know whom our true friends are. We are also more certain than ever that God walks with us."

After cancer, the warrior has to find a "new normal" that fits. Priorities change. Things that seemed immensely important before cancer are now just another thread in the spectacular tapestry of life. Things you took for granted before have now become the focus of your absolute undivided attention.

Friends are more important. So is family. Your physical appearance doesn't matter as much. It's kind of hard to be vain about your looks after you've seen yourself hairless, flabby, and too weak to stand up straight. On the other hand, good eating and good exercise habits have moved up high on the daily to-do list.

Time has a different meaning. It doesn't much matter how long it takes to get to your destination. You spend as much time as you need, and you soak up all the good things on the way. I can get from our house to my office using the Interstate or by taking Scenic Highway along the western shore of Escambia Bay. The trip along the water is five minutes longer. Before cancer, I would never have "wasted" the time to go the long way. The cars cruising along at 45 mph would have frustrated the heck out of me. Now I almost always take the "scenic route."

I found that my job was still exceedingly important to me after cancer, but in a completely different way. Before cancer, my job defined me as a person. When someone asked me, "What do you do?" I never expanded my answer beyond my profession. For 26 years, I was a Naval Officer. For a few weeks I was a university research administrator. Of course, I was also a husband, father, neighbor, and friend—but those titles remained in parentheses in my mind. My job was always in capital letters.

After cancer, I am a husband, father, friend, neighbor—and cancer survivor. I also happen to have a job I really enjoy. It gives me a chance to contribute to my university, my community, and my country. My job is an important part of who I am because it provides me the access to people with whom I enjoy working, talking, and living. And I surely don't take the paycheck lightly. We need it! But what I do for a living is not the complete answer to the question, "What do you do?" In fact, it isn't even the first thing I mention.

Normal isn't what it used be, and I'm glad. It isn't so much that daily life—normal life—is that much different than before cancer. Each morning when I ask the little bird if today is the day, he reminds me to enjoy the routines of life. If I am not enjoying my routine, than I'll alter it until I can enjoy it. Life is far too short to keep plugging away at something you hate. You have two choices. Avoid what you dislike if you can. If not, find a way to fix your attitude.

Don't get the impression that I've become a Pollyanna who can only see the world through rose-colored glasses. Life still has plenty of problems, challenges, and ugliness. I just don't let them ruin my day. Imagine your car radio. You can hit the scan button and catch four-second snatches of all kinds of music. I like lots of different styles—classical, country, classic rock, jazz, blues, and oldies. (You can keep the rap and the Hip-Hop.) They are all available on my radio, but I don't have to listen to them unless I want to. I can slip in a familiar CD if I want. Or I can just turn off the whole thing and enjoy the peace and quiet. Take control and make your own decisions.

SITREP #21

2/18/02

Dear Family, Friends, Shipmates, Classmates, Argonauts, and IHMCers,

Life is good! Today marks four weeks since the final chemo cycle began. So far, no one has grabbed me, thrown me into a recliner, and forced toxic chemicals in my body. Therefore, it also marks the day that I am as free of the drugs as I have been at any time in the last five months. The blood counts should be back to normal in another month, maybe before. I can definitely tell the difference in increased energy and diminished side effects.

We are now entering what can be a scary time for cancer warriors. I had a whole body bone scan on Friday. Tomorrow, I have a series of CT scans. Even though I feel wonderful, it is still a bit frightening to have your future depend on the results of tests for which you can't study. Waiting for the results will be torturous, I'm told. In the best case, I'll get a clean bill of health by the end of the month. Then quarterly check-ups to make sure we catch any abnormal activity in the earliest stages.

Remember that any day in which you learn, laugh, and cry is a good day. I'm trying to make every day a good one. Y'all do the same!

GO USA! Larry

After you've fought the battle and you think maybe you've won, the frightening test week comes. For me it meant whole body bone scans and CT scans of my chest, abdomen, and pelvis. The tests themselves are fairly simple and routine. They don't take an inordinate amount of time.

As a scientist, I found it exceedingly interesting to be on the receiving end of the tracer injection for the bone scans. The stuff is delivered to the Nuclear Medicine clinic in a locked can with "Danger—Radioactive Materials" markings. The technicians wear protective aprons, and your syringe is kept in a lead-shielded tube. You raise your eyebrows when they say, "OK, roll up your sleeve." Do I really need to have my veins become a hazardous materials storage location? But I haven't noticed any ill effects. I don't glow in the dark.

In a different way, the tracer you have to drink for the CT scans has its own side effects. It upsets my stomach and gives me flu-like chills and fatigue for a few hours. All things considered, the tests are easy. You just lie down and let the machines and computers do their thing. There is really no physical discomfort.

But test week is still unbelievably hard. My imagination goes into overdrive as soon as I report to the clinic. Any kind of delay, any re-setting of the machines, or even a cough from the technician immediately triggers irrational fear. Somehow, I think that they know something, and whatever it is, it must be bad news. I know that it is ridiculous. I should be able to think clearly and rationally. Delays, noises, and adjusting the machines are normal parts of the tests. I know that, but somehow it doesn't help me eliminate the fear. I guess it's because so much is riding on the results. And once test day arrives, there isn't a single thing you can do to influence them.

When the tests are over there are several more days of torture while you wait to hear the outcome. I wish the verdict came immediately. But reading the scans takes time and skill. There isn't a green light that flashes up on the computer screen that says "All Clear" or a red banner across the printout with the word "Cancer." Trained specialists interpret the results, and then other experts check them. I understand why there are multiple steps and many checks before results are released. I certainly don't want the wrong answer—either way. My future depends on the test outcome, so I'm glad they take the time to make it as absolutely accurate as possible.

Still, each day in limbo is long and worrisome. I always feel like calling my doctor and shouting, "Don't you all know that reading my tests is the most important thing you've got to do this week?" Somehow I sense they don't share the same urgency that I feel. Nancy and I have a theory that No News is Good News. If something in the test results is suspicious, surely the technicians, radiologists, and doctors will make it high priority. They will show it to the experts right away. On the other hand, we figure that if everything is normal, then it might take a while for the routine report to work through the system. So the longer it takes, the less worried we should be. Too bad it doesn't work that way. Every day of the wait is filled with tension and suspense.

Friday March 1, 2002 is one of the red-letter days in my life. Nancy and I had driven to Dallas for the NCAA Division II Softball Leadoff Classic. It was the big season-opening tournament I had kept my sights on all through the chemotherapy treatment. I made sure Dr. Schneider had my cell phone number, since we expected him to call with the test results any day. I knew he had the preliminary results in his hands, but the final releasing signatures were not yet applied. Until it is official, the patient doesn't get the results. Frustrating, but understandable, I suppose.

Between the Argonauts afternoon and evening games, we returned to the hotel to get out of the chilly drizzle. Usually, you would have to physically drag me away from a softball tournament that included five of the top ten teams in the country. But winter in Dallas just doesn't have much chance of serving up enjoyable softball weather. I was glad to get out of the wind.

Back in our room, the cell phone rang. It was my buddy Les Raske from the Surgery Clinic. He didn't waste any time. He knew how anxious I was to hear the news.

"Hey, Larry. It's Les from Dr. Schneider's office. When can I schedule you to come in to have that mediport removed?"

"Les, does that mean the test results were OK?"

"Well, Bud, only the doctor is allowed to tell you that. But I can tell you that we want to rip out that port. You sure don't need it!"

The cold and the drizzle didn't seem so dismal when I went back to the park for the night games. My Argonaut softball family—Coach Tami and the trainers, players, and parents—helped me celebrate our victory with multiple hot chocolates and a late-night, extra inning win. Even the ice storm that cancelled the rest of the weekend games couldn't dampen our spirits.

Ironically, March 1st was also the day I received the decision on my case from the Navy's Physical Evaluation Board. With hilariously impeccable timing—on the exact same day the doctor told me, "Congratulations, the scans are all clear. You are cancer-free."—my Navy declared me "UNFIT for further duty."

That was actually good news, since it cleared the path for me to once again retire from active duty and go back to work for West Florida. That was my goal in the first place! The Navy placed me on the Temporary Disability Retirement List. Apparently, my particular brand of cancer was an automatic decision for the board. Provided a truck doesn't hit me in the interim, the Navy will do another evaluation 18 months after I went on the temporary list. Then I'll finally achieve my desired spot on the regular role as "United States Navy, Retired."

◆   ◆   ◆

I'm continuously adapting to my "new normal." I am in love with a wonderful wife. I'm a good father. Given the choice, I'll spend my quality time watching fastpitch softball games—on the field as an umpire or in a comfortable chair on the outside of the chain link fence. The sky is bluer, the music is better, the girls are prettier, and the jokes are funnier. I am a Navy retiree, a bad golfer, and a university research administrator. And oh yeah, I'm a cancer survivor.

16

We Are the Lucky Ones

SITREP #22

3/3/02

Dear Family, Friends, Shipmates, Classmates, Argonauts, and IHMCers,

Victory!

Both my bone scans and CAT scans came back clean. There is no evidence of cancer! It looks like we've won this battle.

For all of you who have kept us in your prayers for these last six months, please do one more thing for me. Take a moment to say a quick prayer of thanksgiving with us. Then join us in a toast to modern medical science.

With a vigilant defense and frequent follow-ups, we should be able spot any future intruders early enough to win the skirmishes before they become major battles. Hopefully, no further offensive action will be required. I'll work on strengthening the immune system so that the warfighting force can become peacekeepers instead.

Since I'm finished with Osama the IV stand, I'll have minor surgery Tuesday to remove the mediport from my chest. Then I have an appointment with my oncologist in two weeks to plan the periodic tests and checkups.

It's too bad we are not finished with the real Osama, al Qaeda, and their terrorist counterparts just yet. But that's a bigger war. It will take longer. May our country and our allies have all the strength, courage, and patience needed to keep winning the battles.

GO USA! Larry

After he was declared cancer-free, but before he reached the point that he finally agreed that cancer warriors are truly the lucky ones,

Lance Armstrong went through a drifting period of uncertainty and indecision. Lance calls the phase immediately after cancer Survivorship. It should be a time of celebration, and in many ways, it is. But it can also be exceedingly difficult time. It isn't a simple matter to make the transition from the all-day-every-day existence of the cancer warrior to life as a cancer survivor.

When you are fighting against something that could easily kill you, it is your top priority during every waking minute of every day. Even if you think you are concentrating completely on an unrelated task, cancer is never far from your mind. For more than six months, I never once forgot, even for a split second, that I had cancer. It never slipped my mind. Even in my dreams, my subconscious mind would not forget that I had cancer.

I didn't mind making the cancer battle my number one priority during the chemotherapy and surgery recovery times. But once I was declared cancer-free, I expected to move the whole cancer issue to the "back-burner" of consciousness. Easier said than done. Once you are forced into the habit of looking at every decision, every event, every person, sunset, and raindrop through the cancer lens, it is nearly impossible to see things without considering cancer. This altered view of life, too, becomes a part of the "new normal" for survivors.

I look at this change in outlook as a good thing. If I ever forget that I survived cancer, I may forget to enjoy every day of my precious and short life on earth. I honestly thought I appreciated my life and my family before. I don't think I ever took my good fortune for granted. But now I **really** know what it means to appreciate life!

◆   ◆   ◆

During my half-year as a cancer warrior, I became very self-centered. Even though my contact with the outside world expanded during the battle, and I approached life from a whole new and broader perspective, my expanded universe had me placed firmly in the direct center. In my mind, my world revolved around me. I find it curious that my family communication decreased at a time when I was communicating with more people than ever, and family was more important than ever.

My brothers and I have a long tradition of exchanging monthly family newsletters. The four of us each write three times per year. I don't think I missed a turn in ten years until I started writing cancer SITREPs. Then I missed three times in a row. In retrospect, I think it was because our traditional family newsletters were mostly about the children's activities and our family travels and work travails. I didn't intentionally miss my turn—I just never got around to writing a family newsletter. Probably because it wasn't all about ME, ME, ME.

◆   ◆   ◆

As anxious as the cancer warrior is to declare victory, it isn't a simple matter to say *exactly* when you've won. I declared victory in my 22nd SITREP, but it was probably premature. I won the first battle, but the war goes on. Too often we hear of recurrences. Cancer is an enemy you must defeat, and once beaten, it as a foe for which you must continue to keep watch. The terrorist cells destroyed part of me once. They could re-group and re-attack. Constant vigilance is the price of freedom and good health.

It is a bit frightening to think that something in my lifestyle or background made it possible for cancer to gain a foothold the first time around. I don't think it was a fluke, or that I was simply unlucky. In my case, I am convinced that stress, probably complicated by too much sun and not enough sleep, weakened my immune system and allowed the damaged cells to grow out of control. Along with increased vigilance, I need to make some other lifestyle changes to improve my chances of remaining a *one-time* cancer survivor. In my mind, there's no extra credit for beating it twice.

Fortunately, the cancer experience led me directly to the discovery of the lifestyle changes that hopefully will keep me from repeating the cancer experience. During each chemo cycle, when I reached those good days where my mood swung up to an enjoyable peak, I tried to hang on to that *joie de vivre*. The wonderful mental high is a fragile thing. I quickly discovered that I would lose it if I didn't protect it jealously. Rest, exercise, good food, and mental vacations are my keys to clinging to my newfound love of life. If I short-change any one of those elements, I can quickly forget that I am one of the Lucky Ones.

Sleep is the factor that I found most strongly related to my mood and my attitude. With the possible exception of teenagers and college students who are out of school for the summer, I think American adults are chronically under-rested. It is part of our culture. In fact, most of us brag about how long we can operate on just a few hours of rest per night. In our macho world, it is a mark of prowess to hoot with the owls until the wee hours, and then try to fly with the eagles the next day.

But I've found that my mood and my attitude are directly correlated to the amount of sleep I get. When I was recovering from surgery I was surprised that I could sleep ten hours or more at night and still need a nap in the afternoon. Now that my body is not pouring so much energy into healing, I've settled into seven-and-a-half to eight hours as my optimum night. When I figured out the cost-benefit ratio of setting aside sufficient sleep time, it became an easy decision to define a lifestyle change that put me into bed earlier at night. There is no doubt in my mind that the world would be a kinder, happier, more productive place if everyone got more sleep.

Exercise is the second factor in my quality of life equation. I try for regular, enjoyable workouts. If you push yourself too hard, it isn't fun, and you soon find excuses for not doing it instead of reasons to do it. If you make it a high enough priority, it isn't hard to find 30–60 minutes five times a week. Exercise soon becomes a healthy addiction. It gives you a pleasant high.

For me, one of the biggest benefits of regular vigorous exercise comes at the dinner table. By burning more calories, you can eat more food while still working toward your target weight. Good food is one of the great pleasures of life. I don't believe you have to give up any of your favorite foods to be healthy. You just have to adjust the balance. More fruit and vegetables, less fat and ice cream. More fiber, less refined flour and sugar. If you want to lose weight, it comes down to two simple steps. Eat less. Move around more.

Taking miniature mental vacations is the last key to protecting a joyous mood that I discovered. Whenever possible, I make it a physical vacation as well—an hour on the beach, a ball game, a summer evening concert in the park. But it isn't always possible to get away, even for a few hours. In that case, you can mentally relax through a number of techniques. You can say a prayer, practice deep breathing, meditate, or just daydream. Use whatever method you find to be the most fun and refreshing, because that is probably the one with the biggest benefits for your particular immune system, your productivity, and your attitude.

◆   ◆   ◆

Before cancer I thought that a balanced, even-keel approach to life was the way to go. I figured it was best to level out the inevitable peaks and valleys by not letting myself become overly happy when things were going well and by minimizing problems when life took a sour turn. I reasoned that if I allowed myself to enjoy the good times too much that the subsequent valleys would be even harder to take. I didn't want to set myself up for a fall. Now I have a new approach. I squeeze every drop of happiness I can out of the good days. Life's too short not to ride the roller coaster all the way to the top.

Of course there will be valleys to go with the peaks. As Colin Powell says, "You can't slay dragons every day. Some days the dragons win." But I've got the keys to shortening the bad days. Two full nights of sleep and two good workouts will always put the bounce back in my stride and the spark back in my eye. A mini-vacation increases my energy level, and I can sustain that energy longer by cutting out the Krispy Kremes and adding extra vegetables and fruits in the diet. The obstacles that seemed overwhelming earlier in the week are now manageable. The stumbling blocks become stepping-stones.

SITREP #23 (The LAST One)

3/20/02

Dear Family, Friends, Shipmates, Classmates, Argonauts, and IHMCers,

On this first day of Spring, as the world thinks about the new life that comes with the changing of the seasons, it is appropriate that I close the cancer chapter that you all helped me survive during the last fall and winter. Our e-mail exchange has been a tremendous morale booster for the Lovely Nurse Nancy and me. Just because I stop broadcasting SITREPs, please don't stop corresponding. We love hearing from you!

I am now officially a survivor, although one who will require regular checks, scans, and tests for the next several years. My appointment with the oncologist last week was more victory celebration than medical visit. I feel absolutely wonderful, even though the blood counts are just now returning to the lower end of the "normal" range. Now I will try to put my cancer concerns "on the back burner," because life is proceeding at full speed.

- We are now the proud owners of a new home in Pace, Florida, having closed last Friday.

- The Navy bureaucracy decided to allow me to retire (again).

- I will resume my job as the University of West Florida's Sponsored Research Executive on April 1st. (No Fool's jokes, please!)

- We will move our household goods from Louisiana to Florida in April (even though the LA house STILL hasn't closed).

- I'm having a blast umpiring college fastpitch softball during the numerous Spring Break tournaments in Pensacola.

I wish there was a way to teach people how to feel as good as I feel without going through what I had to go through to get here. I'll have to work on that.

GO USA! Larry

By the time I reached the mid-point of chemotherapy, I was pretty well convinced that cancer warriors really are The Lucky Ones. Even without knowing if I was going to join the millions of survivors, I was ready to admit that my life—however long it was going to last—had changed for the better. I certainly believed that I had appreciated life before cancer, but I really didn't have a clue how to really enjoy every day, every minute.

I don't want to give the impression that I think life is perfect. It's just that I've discovered that with the right attitude, it is entirely possible to enjoy even the unpleasant experiences life shoves your way. If it's hot and humid when I head out for my lunchtime walk, I only need to remind myself that you have to be alive to sweat. The ball game was rained out? No problem. Any weather is enjoyable if your alternative is no weather at all. Likewise, problems in any particular phase of life are just challenges that can be tackled because you're alive to tackle them. Everything works out in the end. If it hasn't worked out yet, then it isn't the end.

I can tell you that this plus side of cancer is not confined only to those of us who survive. I read a number of stories in which friends and family members say that their loved one's appreciation for life increased markedly, even as the quality of that life decreased rapidly. You often hear that someone who succumbed to cancer fought a heroic battle. I don't think people are just saying nice things about the deceased. The warriors found that fighting a good fight to the end helps them face the frightening battle. Anyone can be a hero—if there's no other choice.

◆   ◆   ◆

A shipmate of mine a dozen years ago was one of these heroes. Having survived cancer helped me finally understand and cope with his death. My good friend was struck down at the peak of life. A fine young officer in his early thirties, he had a terrific family—three handsome, polite, and smart young sons and a wonderful wife. He was a devout man with a great sense of humor. His distinctive laugh lightened the day for everyone on the ship.

One night when we were at sea in the Mediterranean he suffered a seizure and fell in the passageway. The doc didn't like what he saw in his vital signs, so he arranged to have him flown to a military hospital in Germany for tests.

We were all shocked to find out he had a rapidly growing malignant brain tumor. Surgery stabilized his condition, but there was no doubt that he would soon lose his battle. Months later, when his count of days was hastily dwindling, we sat on my back deck and talked for hours as we nursed a couple of beers. He told me then that he thought he was a very lucky man. I thought he was just putting up a brave front. (Actually, at the time I really wondered if the tumor had affected his judgment—although he seemed perfectly cogent.) It didn't seem possible that his irrepressible spirit and positive attitude had survived all the bad news he had absorbed. Now, I know that he really meant it when he said he considered himself lucky.

What was it that made my dying friend a lucky man? He explained that he thought he was blessed to have the time to take care of his wife's security, set up his sons' educational plans, and to say farewell to all his friends and family. Yes, he was angry that he would miss so much of life, but he figured he was much better off than someone who left home one morning without kissing his kids goodbye and was killed on the highway before he was able to walk through his door again that evening.

◆   ◆   ◆

Family ties are strengthened and reinforced during the cancer battle. Even broken ties can be re-tied. Some cancer warriors are blessed, as I am, with large families of siblings, parents, children, cousins and in-laws. But I don't restrict my family to the usual definition requiring ties of blood or marriage. Shared interests and experiences make family members of a wide range of people. I was overwhelmed by the kindness and concern from my classmates from the U.S. Naval Academy Class of 1975. Softball friends became part of my extended family. Our Navy friends were terrific—especially in how they made sure that Nancy was getting all the help and emotional support she needed. The wonderful people of the Naval Oceanographic Office—my professional family for three years—showed me that I was still a welcome part of the NAVO team.

To paraphrase Lance Armstrong, once you hear the words, "You have cancer," and think "I'm going to die," you're in the cancer community. Once you're in it, you never leave. Cancer warriors, both new fighters and old survivors, become part of your extended family. For survivors, many of us feel something that's been called "the obligation of the cured." We want to give something back to the community that helped us win our victory. Not surprisingly, a large percentage of cancer fundraiser volunteers are former warriors and their families.

I personally drew great strength from other cancer warriors and survivors. I feel I can best meet the obligation of the cured by sharing my cancer experience with others. As early as the middle of my chemo, I began to get calls and emails from friends who thought that I could help someone they knew who was fighting the battle. I always say yes. I will write, call, or email. Hopefully, I can help another cancer warrior as much as former survivors helped me.

◆   ◆   ◆

I am certainly not the first cancer warrior to feel compelled to write about my experience. During the first weeks of my war, I was inspired by a handful of books by survivors. They gave me courage and confidence. I want to add to the list. I also want to try to share the lesson I learned during the battle. As I said in my final SITREP, I'd like to be able to tell people how to feel as good as I feel right now—without going through what I had to go through to get there.

It can be done. And it isn't hard. In fact, it is simple. But like the "eat less and move around more" weight loss system, there are no magic elixirs or secret combinations of ingredients. In fact, the keys to reaching a wonderful enjoyment of everyday life are downright trite and boring. They are pretty much the same things you've heard preached at you from the time your mother stopped talking baby talk in your face.

- Eat right.
- Don't smoke.
- Exercise.
- Get more sleep than you have been getting.
- Relax.
- Stop and smell the flowers.
- Smile.
- Follow the Golden Rule (the one that begins "Do unto others…" not the "Them that has the gold…" version.)
- Say your prayers.
- Use sunscreen.

- Keep an imaginary bird on your shoulder. Ask it if today is the last day of your life. Act accordingly.

- Follow Jim Valvano's advice: laugh, learn, and cry—every day.

Afterword

The idea for this book came from the logical convergence of two separate and different writing streams. The first series of writings were the Situation Reports that Nancy and I sent to our friends. I started composing the first one during the turmoil of September 11th. Many people around the world felt compelled to record their feelings in the wake of the tragedy. I felt a strong desire to capture my deep conviction that America would rise taller than ever. Somehow, during that tumultuous week of mid-September, deep in my emotionally taxed mind, I tied my own cancer battle to the war on terrorism.

In light of the cataclysmic events in Washington, New York, and Pennsylvania, my personal situation should have dwindled to insignificance. Instead, the linkage in my mind between the two wars made me feel that it was more important than ever to be strong and courageous in my own small world. The character embodied in George Bush, Rudy Giuliani, and thousands of unnamed heroes fed my determination to fight my battle to the best of my ability.

Another motive of my SITREP series was to reassure our friends and family and give them something good on which to focus their concentration. I knew people would worry about me anyway. It isn't that I didn't want anyone to worry. On the contrary, I wanted them to worry about me, think about me, and pray for me constantly. But somehow, I wanted people to have an optimistic and confident outlook.

I've always believed that pessimists and optimists are **both** right—that is, they both will get pretty much what they expect. I think I unconsciously wanted the prayers on my behalf to be prayed with positive words ("God, give Larry strength to beat this bugger.") I didn't even want a negative thought ("God, don't let Larry die.") to cross anyone's mind. Does God care? I don't think so. But does it make sense anyway? Maybe.

The SITREPs became a popular, if irregular, addition to a lot of electronic mail boxes. If I let too much time pass between writings, Nancy and I would get calls and e-mails asking for an update. I think people just felt relieved to hear that everything was proceeding according to plan. On our end, Nancy and I looked forward to the flood of replies that came back to us each time. Our worldwide support network was a vital part of our existence in a challenging time.

♦   ♦   ♦

The second writing stream began a few weeks after surgery. A friend suggested journaling as an exercise to pass time, to provide mental stimulation, and to combat worry and depression. The concept behind writing a journal is to keep a private diary in which to record thoughts, worries, ideas, concerns, and random flights of fancy. I started writing entries in my laptop under a Journal file.

As I read back over the first few entries, it soon became very clear to me that I was writing not for myself, but for others. I felt like I could express some thoughts and experiences for other cancer warriors, their friends, and their families. The Journal file quickly became a disorganized collection of thoughts and stories that I thought might be useful in a book about my personal war.

When I realized I had won the battle, I wondered if there was a way for my friends to feel as good about life as I did—without going through the horrors I underwent. I really don't think you can join the legion of Lucky Ones without getting into the arena first. Still, I firmly believe that some of the lessons I learned can translate into a better quality of life for anyone willing to make the small investment in taking better care of their physical, mental, and emotional health. I would like everyone to share my outlook on life. It's fun!

♦   ♦   ♦

The two writing streams converged when a number of friends complimented the SITREP e-mails. Many times they told me, "You ought to write a book."

At first I said, "Maybe I will."

Eventually the answer changed to, "I'm working on it."

Now I can say, "I did!"

0-595-24101-8